THE PERFECT 10 DETOX

A plant-based program designed to improve your health and lose waste in ten days

Angela Bentley-Henry, M.Ed.

Copyright © [2025] by [Angela Bentley-Henry, M.Ed.]

All rights reserved.

No portion of this book may be reproduced in any form without written permission from the publisher or author, except as permitted by U.S. copyright law.

This publication is designed to provide educational information in regard to the subject matter covered. It is sold with the understanding that neither the author nor the publisher is engaged in rendering legal, health, nutrition, or other professional services. While the publisher and author have used their best efforts in preparing this book, they make no representations or warranties with respect to the accuracy or completeness of the contents of this book and specifically disclaim any implied warranties of merchantability for a particular purpose. No warranty may be created or extended by sales representatives or written sales materials. The advice and strategies contained herein may not be suitable for your situation. You should consult with a professional when appropriate. The author is not a doctor, they cannot heal, diagnose, or cure you of anything. You assume all risk for any nutritional or fitness information you engage in. Neither the publisher nor the author shall be liable for any loss of profit or any other commercial damages, including but not limited to special, incidental, consequential, personal, or other damages.

Book Front and Back Cover by [Angela Bentley-Henry, M.Ed.]

Table of Contents

- _Toc207027576Chapter 1 The Choice Is Yours 2
- Chapter 2: Results Don't Lie 7
- Chapter3: UnderstandingtheDetoxProcess 18
- Chapter 4: The Perfect 10 Core Principles 30
- Chapter 5: The Perfect 10 Phase 1 54
- Chapter 6: The Perfect 10 Phase 2 65
- Chapter 7: The Perfect 10 Phase 3 74
- Chapter 8: Where Should I Start? 82
- Chapter 9: My Journey to Plants 87
- Chapter 10: There Are No Dumb Questions 102
- Chapter 11: Join The Challenge 112
- Chapter 12: Recipes, Food Ideas, and Tips 116
- Chapter 13: What's Now? 149
- About The Author 156
- Citations 160

The Choice Is Yours

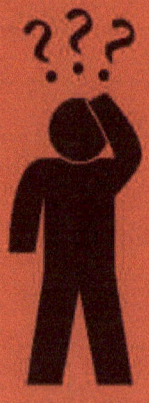

Chapter 1
The Choice Is Yours

I can't remember where I heard this or read this, but it has stuck with me for quite some time now:

IF YOU WANT TO BE HEALTHY, THEN LIVE HEALTHY!

A simple concept, but it changed me. Whatever you are after, stop saying that's what you want and just start living like you have already achieved it.

The choice is yours.

Think about it. Have you ever been walking in a park and seen someone cycling, and thought to yourself, "I want to get into riding my bike more?" You think it, you say it, but nothing comes of it because often in life we complicate what doesn't need to be complicated.

"Do you want to be a cyclist?" Then go outside and start cycling! Consistently do it, and eventually, you will get good at it and be a "cyclist".

The choice is yours.

"Do you want to complete a nutritional challenge?" Find one that aligns with your goals. Do your research, buy the food, and eat accordingly.

The choice is yours.

Those are just two examples, but I'm sure you get the idea, don't stop at the thinking, and saying of a goal, jump right into the doing.

The choice is yours.

Before we dive into The Perfect 10 Detox program, there are two things I want to say:

Number 1, thank you for picking up a copy of this book, this shows me you are ready to stop talking and ready to start doing.

Number 2, **food is a powerful medicine,** especially plant food, so before you begin any nutritional program, please consult with your doctor or physician.

Arguably 8 out of the top 10 leading causes of death in the United States are related to lifestyle. According to the Centers for Disease Control and Prevention (CDC), as of October 25, 2024 review, the top leading causes of death (ranking and number of deaths) were:

1. **Heart disease: 702,880**
2. **Cancer: 608,371**
3. COVID-19: 186,552
4. Accidents (unintentional injuries): 227,039
5. **Stroke (cerebrovascular diseases): 165,393**
6. **Chronic lower respiratory diseases: 147,382**
7. **Alzheimer's disease: 120,122**
8. **Diabetes: 101,209**
9. **Chronic liver disease and cirrhosis: 54,803**
10. **Nephritis, nephrotic syndrome, and nephrosis: 57,937**

(https://www.cdc.gov/nchs/fastats/leading-causes-of-death.htm)

Lifestyle diseases are those diseases that are not communicable, or contagious and are often caused by the lifestyle choices that a person makes. Those lifestyle choices, or risk factors, may include excessive tobacco use, an unhealthy nutritional diet, lack of physical activity, excessive alcohol use, consumption of excessive sugary, salty, an fatty foods and drinks, and being overweight or obese.

Knowing that so much concerning our health is preventable and reversible makes my first thought be, "Why don't we just change our lifestyle?". You know, change the way we eat, change the way we think, change our daily habits. Live the lifestyle that produces the life we desire.

My second thought is, "How can I help others with the knowledge that I know?"

I could sit here and make myself sound perfect and as if I have all the answers, but that would be a lie. You see it took a series of drastic wake-up calls for me to finally change my habits. So, "Do these experiences make me an expert?" No. Not at all. They make me a testimony. It also makes me have a strong desire to help others experience health, experience the body they desire, and ultimately live a higher quality of life. "Don't believe me?" I get it, the idea that consuming plants and lifestyle changes can transform our health is a far-fetched thought for many.

Ultimately, the fate of your health is in your own hands.

The choice is yours.

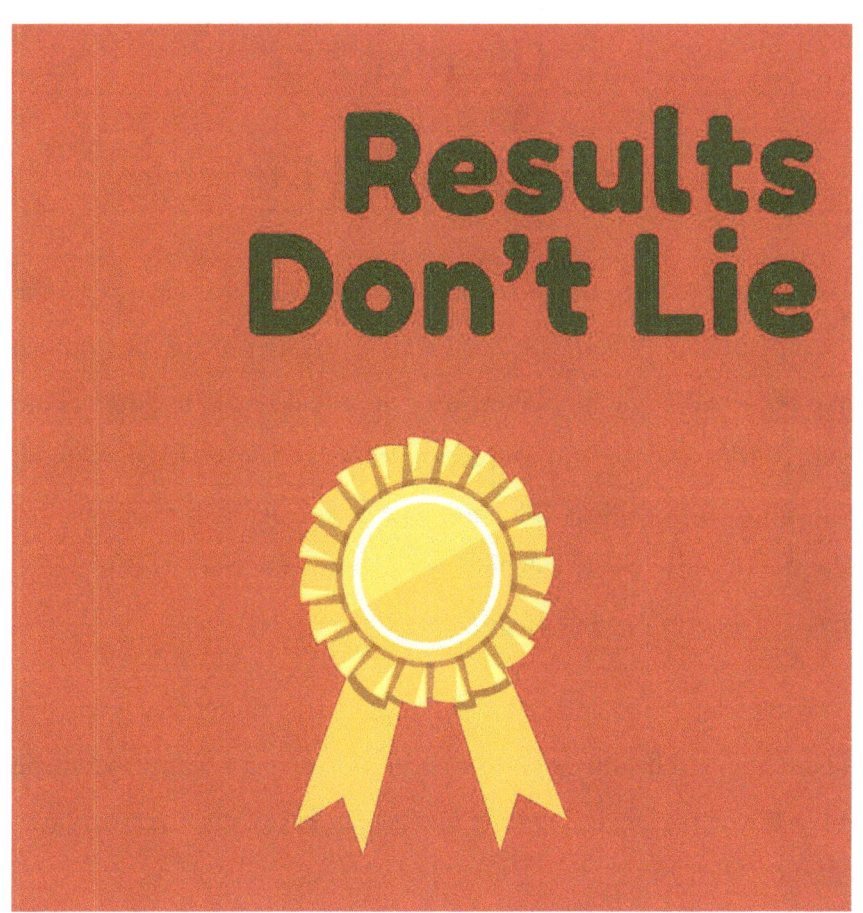

Chapter 2

Results Don't Lie

Many of you reading this book and embarking on this cleanse, are in a health situation where you need results quickly, or maybe you just have been making some unhealthy choices and need to get back on track. Either way, it's important to note that knowledge without application is worthless. Meaning, what you learn throughout this cleanse will only be as valuable as the application of its principles. That will determine your results.

Speaking from personal experience, I was not applying the knowledge of detoxing and healthy eating back in 2015 when I was pre-diabetic and overweight, nor in the time leading up to my discovery of heart issues in April 2022.

I was not taking care of myself properly and my body just chose those times in my life to reveal all the damage. Yes, it can be scary. Yes, it can be challenging. But, "What is the alternative?", a low quality of life, plagued with health issues and unhealthy symptoms. No, thank you! That will not be my story. And, it does not have to be yours either.

It's not enough for a coach or author to say that a particular program has worked, "for me", using the principles of a program to benefit large groups of people, is a much better way to evaluate if a program works. Well, that's exactly what I did with The Perfect 10 Detox Private Group.

I have used The Perfect 10 principles to nutritionally coach individuals one-on-one as well as host large group challenges for quite some time now. I would like to thank each participant and client who has been willing to share their story and experiences while working with me and completing the detox.

Below I will share with you some of the positives that clients have experienced following The Perfect 10 Detox program.

Here are some of their success stories:

Testimonial 1

I haven't checked the scale; however, I definitely feel the difference and my clothes fit differently. My wife said that I lost some stomach fat. The first 5 days I felt lighter with more energy. It {The Detox program} has helped with the bloating and pain I have been having in my ankle and Achilles. I don't know if it is waste loss or not eating all the other stuff {junk foods}. My joints feel better.

-Shaquille H.

Testimonial 2

Seven days ago, I started working with Coach Bentley-Henry to kick start my weight loss journey weighing in at 214.8 pounds. I've been on this cycle of losing weight and gaining weight for about 10 years now and the most difficult part is always finding something I'm comfortable with and will show results to keep my head in the game.

Week one has been all about a reset, fruit only (Phase 3). This was a clean cut from nothing but Coca-Cola all day and all the fun, fast, sugary foods. I was nervous about the sugar withdrawals and my soda addiction (it was fierce).

I was surprised that eating fruits would be filling and help with the sweet cravings. For the most part, mentally, I managed well, but I had moments of cravings for unhealthy food choices like pizza, burgers, and chips. But I was not hungry, I just wanted the flavor.

I only had a headache one day near the beginning but after reviewing my fruit and water intake with my coach, it was apparent I was not drinking enough water and going too long between eating (busy at work).

Reflecting on the experience this week – the most difficult part was changing my behavior of being intentional about always having fruit and water readily accessible. However, it wasn't hard to do at all. I just had to be mindful and intentional about what I was purchasing and planning.

The best part was the personal coaching, tracking the progress, and celebrating each progress.

The coach was consistently monitoring my intake and coaching me on what to focus on. More water intake, being careful of salt, and which fruits help with what I needed personally in my journey. I could share what I was struggling with such as forgetting my food at home, cravings, difficulty drinking water, and fighting the mental cravings of food. I was never hungry. I'm thankful for that because I know that is my weak point. I'll go through a drive-through and indulge. It's important to note that it wasn't entirely difficult to go out to eat or continue with normal outings that involve food. Coach helped me work through those moments on how to prepare myself and it worked out beautifully.

My starting weight was 214.8 pounds. My ending weight of week one was 208.8 pounds for a total loss of 6 pounds.

My size 18 pants were too loose yesterday; that made me feel good. I was so happy. When people noticed I had dropped some weight, one person pointed out that my face looked different (slimmer).

Week 2, let's go!

Christina D

Testimonial 3

It was definitely an enlightening experience. It aided with getting my gut regulated after months of me getting off course stemming from the holidays.

Pros: Mental awareness and clarity, overall waste elimination, new fun recipes, and energy boosts. {At first} I had to slow down the intensity of working out as my intake shifted, but Angela provided me with direction. Once I followed {her directions} I was able to sustain my weights again.

Cons: Headaches and side effects from detoxing (which I expected as I drink an excessive amount of coffee).

Danille H.

Testimonial 4

I'm loving it…I feel so good and I have lost 5 pounds. I have been getting rid of waste for sure and gaining so much energy and it feels good. No more brain fog, and I'm super focused.

-Waynetta P.

Testimonial 5

I got up to 226 lbs. and said ain't no way I'm going to be this big. I started with the detox mindset, thanks to Angela Bentley-Henry. My biggest and best meal of the day is breakfast so I replaced my breakfast with an all-natural smoothie with no sugar added! This is week 3 for me and I'm 216. I'm loving this new healthy way of eating lifestyle. What works for me may not work for you, but it's more mental than anything with me.

-Shawana S.

Testimonial 6

Good morning, after the sea moss gel and the gummies my blood pressure is perfect, it used to be high.

-Brandon G.

Testimonial 7

Enjoyed this, it truly jumped-started my thought process and choices when it comes to what I eat. Thanks to everyone for sharing.

Rochelle L-B.

Testimonial 8

I'm down 5 pounds. I'm sleeping better. I'm thankful for doing this challenge and last month's challenge. It was well worth it. Thanks, Angela Bentley-Henry.

-Arlene S.

Testimonial 9

This was an eye-opening experience for me. Proud of what I've learned and accomplished throughout this process. Thank you to everyone and a special thank you to Angela Bentley-Henry for creating this challenge. Looking forward to the next!

This challenge has helped me to think about how food choices affect my health. I've been eating more fresh fruits and vegetables. I feel better, have more energy, and sleep better. I've been taking fresh squeezed juices and smoothies with me while I'm on the go. Thanks, Angela Bentley-Henry for the challenge. It was just what I needed. I appreciate you sharing your knowledge.

-Patty H.

Testimonial 10

So, the thing I've noticed lately is I have chronic dry lips. I've done everything that I can to moisturize them and I drink mostly water all the time. They never smooth out, they're always dry somehow. But eating all these fruits seems to have done the trick. They are not nearly as dry as they have been in a very long time.

-Barbara S.

Testimonial 11

In loving memory of Lynn Driver (Educator, Sports Analyst, Friend)

It took me over three years to start loving myself again! After suffering from depression for over two years, I was wondering why God kept waking me up. I began to realize through all the pain I suffered, I lost the most important relationship in my life, ME! I told myself that for me to change, I must do things that I have never done before.

So, I began my journey to meet the most important person in my life. Myself. It was at that moment my journey began. First, I wanted to be obedient to the teachings of someone who I knew would place the responsibility on me, and me only. At the same time show great support and understanding. I contacted Angela Henry. I knew she was a no-nonsense, put-your-head-down, and grind-type of person.

Since Angela became my health coach and mentor, my life has been overflowing with happiness and confidence. On June 14th, my blood pressure was 160/100 and I weighed 473 pounds. I followed Angela's plan for health and weight loss and by June 21st, I weighed 463 pounds. Amazingly my blood pressure went down to 112/70. I continued following the plan for another 5 days, and by June 27th, I dropped an additional 15 pounds to 448. During my journey, Angela introduced me to a support group that has shown me so much love and support. As a result of my weight loss, I can now walk around much faster with better endurance. Thanks to Angela and plants, I will soon meet the most important person in my life. Myself!

These are just a handful of the amazing results that have come out of The Perfect 10 Detox program.

Results don't lie!

I'm excited to be there to hear your success story once you complete The Perfect 10 Detox too!

I shared these personal triumphs of others with you, and will share my personal story in detail with you (later in this book) for four reasons:

1. It's time for you to get real with yourself and evaluate your current condition.
2. It's time to apply the knowledge and guidelines that you are about to learn to begin, "your success story".
3. Lifestyle diseases and a low quality of life do not have to be your fate. The choice is yours.
4. **Results don't lie!**

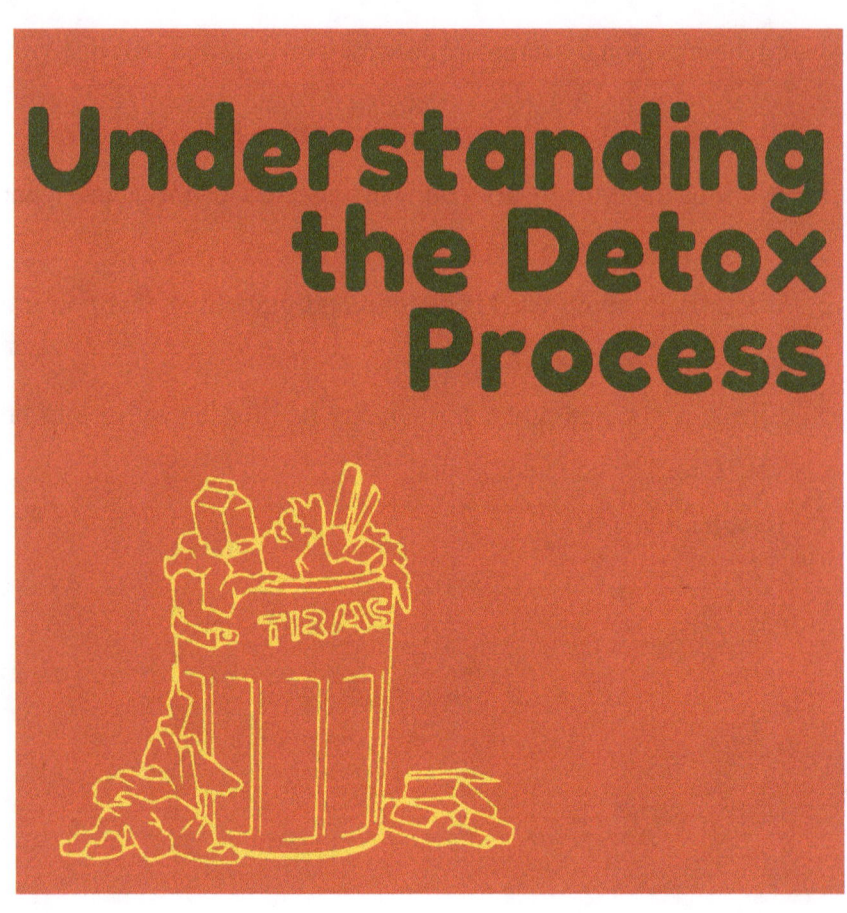

Chapter 3

Understanding the Detox Process

"Who was this cleanse designed for?" When starting any type of nutritional program or challenge, it's important to self-evaluate. Ask yourself, "What is my goal? What am I currently dealing with? What do I want to change about my health?"

After coaching group challenges using The Perfect 10 system, I have listed common reasons and issues that those who participate in the detox are dealing with:

- Low Energy
- Brain Fog
- Excess Belly Fat
- Constipation
- Overweight
- Acne
- Sleeping Issues
- Hypertension
- High Cholesterol
- Hormonal Imbalances
- Erectile Dysfunction
- Bad Smelling Urine
- Insulin Resistance

"Are you having any of these issues?" If you answered yes, then you are in the right place.

The Perfect 10 Detox system is designed for all levels of health. Whether this is your first cleanse or tenth. The Perfect 10 system will be a good fit for you.

The purpose of "The Perfect 10 program" is to eliminate toxins and make healthier the body's major elimination pathways, which allows the body to heal itself, and maintain or reach its ideal weight.

This is not a diet to follow every day for life.

Before I get into why we need to cleanse, how we eliminate, and ways to improve the detoxification process, an important fact to note is that our body detoxes and cleanses itself on its own. It does not necessarily "need" a special supplement, tea, or food to do so. Our bodies only need time and an abundance of nutrients to get the job done.

You may be wondering, "What a cleanse or detox is?", or even "What is a toxin?" Throughout this book, I will be using those terms very often, so let me explain them first.

The terms cleanse and detox are often used interchangeably. But there is a difference. Cleanses tend to require a shorter amount of commitment time. Whereas detoxes typically take longer and cleanse the body on a deeper level. Out of the two, detoxes tend to be more comprehensive in their approach, but both are aimed at eliminating toxins for healing and waste loss. For the sake of this book, and The Perfect 10 program, those terms will be used interchangeably.

Toxins are harmful substances to your body. Toxins can be absorbed in the body by what you put on your skin, what you inhale, and by what is consumed by mouth.

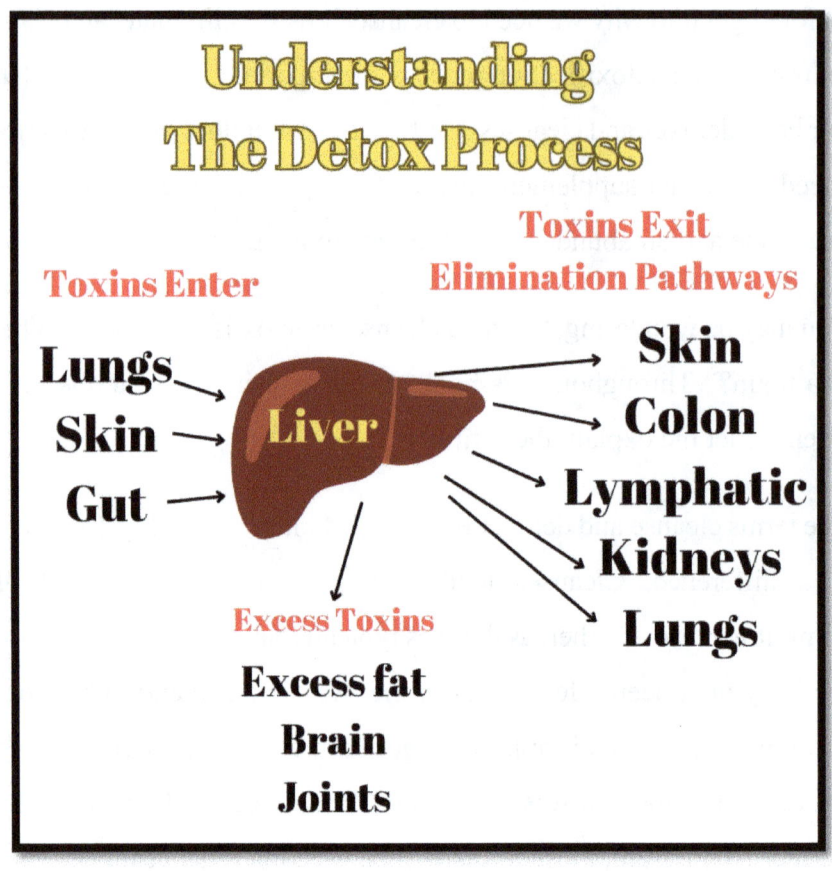

There are 3 ways toxins penetrate our bodies:

1. Through the lungs - pollution, smog, smoke, mold, fumes, basically anything we breathe in.
2. Through the skin - lotion, creams, soaps, toiletries, cosmetics, sprays, basically anything put on the skin.
3. Through the gut - chemicals in food, pesticides, add sugar foods and liquids, processed junk foods, basically anything we ingest (eat or drink).

Once toxins enter our body, and aren't removed, this is where disease, weight issues, and health issues arise.

Our bodies remove these toxins through what's known as elimination pathways or detoxification pathways.

Here are 7 of the major elimination pathways:

1. Liver
2. Skin
3. Kidneys
4. Colon
5. Lungs
6. Lymphatic
7. Emotions

Each pathway has a specific job to do in keeping our body clean. The method by which these pathways are eliminated can look like the following:

1. Liver
- ✓ All toxins filter through the liver. It is the primary filtration system in the body. It is arguably the most important organ for eliminating toxins. As the liver filters, it passes along or moves the toxins to one of the other major pathways.

2. Skin
- ✓ Toxins are eliminated as rashes or acne.

3. **Eyes and Nose**
   ✓ Toxins are eliminated as discharge, pink eye, and sinus drainage.

4. **Kidneys**
   ✓ Toxins are eliminated as urine.

5. **Colon**
   ✓ Toxins are eliminated as solid waste.

6. **Lungs**
   ✓ Toxins are eliminated by breathing or coughing.

7. **Lymphatic**
   ✓ Toxins are eliminated in lymph nodes.
   ✓ Lymph fluid carrying toxins will build up and cause swelling if it is not drained in some way.
   ✓ Lymph nodes are located in the neck, armpit, chest, abdomen (belly), and groin area. There are many lymph node locations.

8. **Emotions**
   ✓ As a person cleanses toxins from their physical toxins, the more undealt with emotions on a spiritual and emotional level may surface. Emotions such as frustration, anger, resentment, depression, anxiety, and even fear are often released during a cleanse.

✓ These toxins can be eliminated through laughter, crying, prayer, meditation, and even journaling.

Excessive accumulation of toxins lead to blocked and unhealthy pathways as well as an unhealthy liver. The blocked and unhealthy pathways cause toxins to not be able to be eliminated from the body.

The combination of the body's liver not being able to filter properly, and the blocked or unhealthy pathways results in the excessive toxins being sent to:

1. Fat Cells
2. The Brain
3. Joints
    - Fat cells full of toxins = weight gain, diabetes, etc.
    - The brain full of toxins = brain fog, dementia, Alzheimer's, stroke, nerve issues, etc.
    - Joints full of toxins = inflammation

Ever wonder why you have a hard time losing weight? Or why your health issues don't seem to be improving? This is why! Your pathways are blocked or unhealthy.

This is why a cleanse or detox is necessary. It helps to keep and attain healthy pathways so they can do their job in eliminating those unwanted substances.

This is not a dietary guideline to follow for life.

Cleansing sometimes comes with unwanted symptoms. These are referred to as, detox symptoms. Detox symptoms can vary depending on which elimination pathways of your body are unhealthy or blocked.

Detox symptoms are also often caused by preexisting inflammation in the body. Inflammation is the process of notifying the immune system that it needs to defend the body from various bacteria, viruses, and injuries. This process or virus can come with unwanted symptoms.

It's important to provide examples of how inflammation may show itself as it's a term used quite often.

- When you have an ear infection and run a fever, that's inflammation.
- When you eat something heavily processed or old and get diarrhea, that's inflammation.
- You have swelling in your knee after jumping, that's inflammation.

Here are some examples of detoxification symptoms and inflammation you may experience during a cleanse:

- Skin = Acne and rashes
- Eyes and Nose = Sinus congestion, pink eye

- Kidneys = Kidney pains or infections, bladder infections
- Colon = Constipation, difficulty losing weight
- Lungs = Congestion
- Lymphatic = Lymph nodes swell, sore throat, flu-like symptoms
- Emotions = Crying, laughter, sadness

Although these symptoms are uncomfortable, know that these symptoms mean your body is eliminating and healing those specific pathways. Some refer to this stage as the "healing crisis".

In addition to implementing The Perfect 10 Detox program, these strategies will assist in opening the elimination pathways:

1. Skin and Lymphatic Pathway

<u>Sweating</u>

1. Will help open skin and lymph pathways.
   - Great ways to sweat include hot yoga, sauna, exercise, or even wearing a sauna suit.

<u>Dry Brushing</u>

- Will open up the pores on your skin, which helps unblock the skin and lymph pathways.

- Locations to dry brush include under your armpits, the sides of your throat, and the groin area. These areas have a lot of lymph nodes.
- Loofah.
- Used in shower. Can be purchased online or at local stores.
- Used to scrub the armpit area, the groin area, and the sides of the throat.

<u>Jumping (rebounding)</u>

- The motion of bouncing up and down stimulates the immune system and helps your body get rid of toxins through increased lymph drainage.

2. **Liver Pathway**
   - Stay hydrated.
   - Eat, blend, or juice greens -especially cruciferous vegetables such as broccoli, cauliflower, and arugula.

3. **Colon Pathway**
   - Consuming a fiber-rich diet (fruits and vegetables).
   - Abdomen massage.
   - Defecate.

4. **Kidney Pathway**
   - Stay hydrated.
   - Do not hold your urine in.
   - Increase consumption of fruits and herbs like cilantro and parsley.

5. **Lungs Pathway**
    - Increase Vitamin D-rich foods.
    - Mushrooms, oranges, spinach, and bananas.
    - Increase anti-inflammatory foods and drinks.
    - Berries, broccoli, turmeric, and green tea.
    - Deep breathing and laughing.
    - Spend more time outside around trees for fresh air.
6. **Eyes and Nose Pathway**
    - Apply a warm compress to the nose area. This may help open up the nasal passage from the outside.
7. **Emotions**
    - Take time to address your thoughts and feelings.
    - Journal, exercise, pray, meditate, cry, and laugh.

The Perfect 10 Core Principles

Chapter 4

The Perfect 10 Core Principles

The Perfect 10 Detox program is a 10-day, plant-based, 3-phase program. Its goal is to cleanse the body on a cellular level in an effort to remove waste (weight that should not be there), improve lifestyle diseases, such as diabetes, hypertension, high cholesterol, low energy, excess belly fat, brain fog, and kickstart any long-term nutritional plan.

What makes The Perfect 10 special is there is a proven formula in place for success that has been used and tested over time with many groups of people.

The core principles, known as "The Perfect 10," are what aid the body in the detoxification process:

The Perfect 10

1. High Water Content Fruits
2. Non-Starchy Vegetables
3. Herbs
4. Low Fat
5. High Fiber
6. No Added Sugar, Oils, or Salt
7. Hydration
8. Sea Vegetables
9. Movement/Sleep
10. Digestion Times

1. **High Water Content Fruits**

   These are fruits that have 80% water content or higher. They tend to be low fat and high fiber. This category also includes botanical fruits. Botanical fruits are "fruits" that are usually categorized as vegetables.

   The water content in fruits helps our bodies stay properly hydrated.

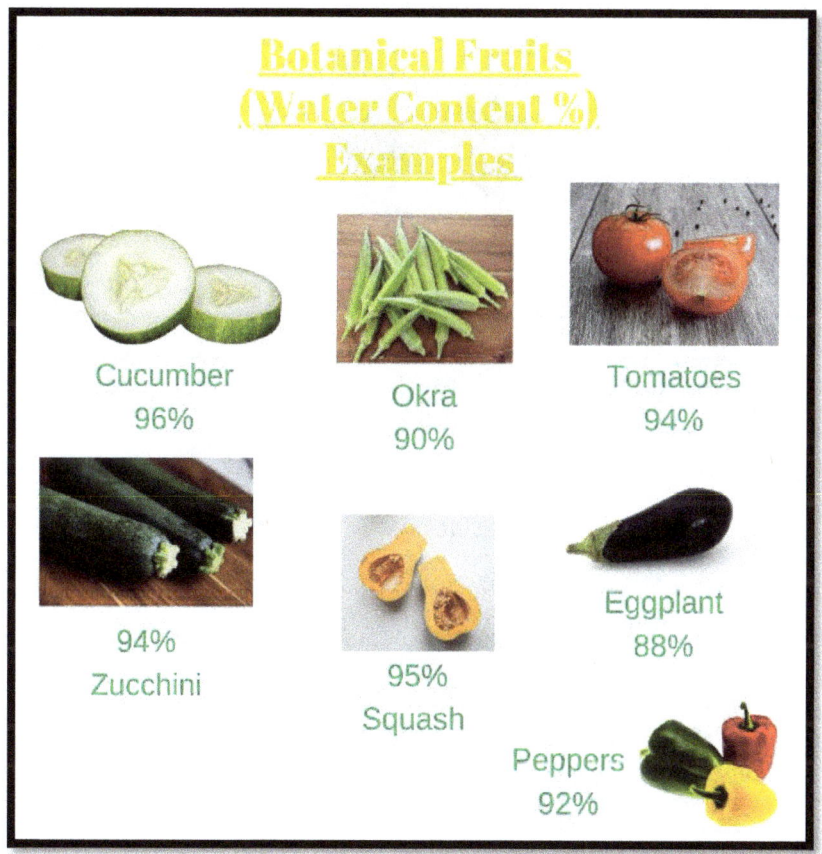

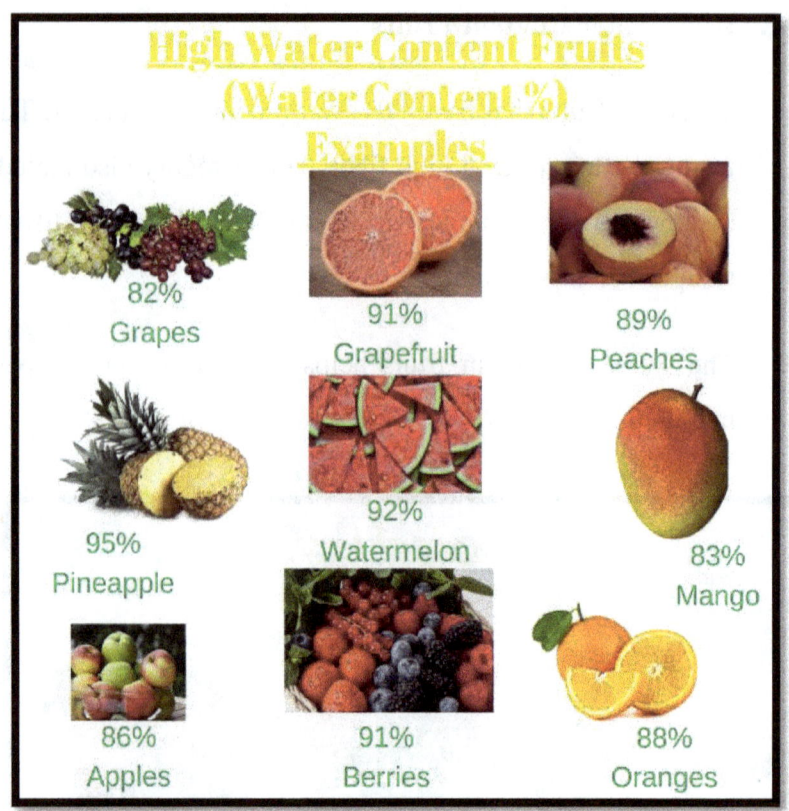

2. **Non-Starchy Vegetables**

These vegetables are full of vitamins, minerals, fiber, and phytonutrients. Non-starchy vegetables are low-calorie. A good portion of the non-starchy vegetables that will be consumed will be greens.

Non-Starchy Vegetables	Vitamins/Minerals
Asparagus	B9, A, B1, B2, B6, and C

	Potassium, Copper, Calcium, Iron, and Phosphorus
Broccoli	A, B6, B12, D, E, and K, Calcium, Iron, Phosphorous, Potassium, Zinc, Thiamin, Riboflavin, Niacin, Manganese
Romaine Lettuce	C, K, A, Folate, Phosphorus, Calcium, Magnesium, Potassium
Green Cabbage, cooked	K, C, B6, Folate, Manganese, Calcium, Potassium, Magnesium
Cauliflower	C, K, Calcium, Potassium, Magnesium, Folate
Spinach	C, A, K, Iron, Folate, Calcium, Potassium, Magnesium
Kale	A, C, K, Folate, Lutein, Phosphorus, Potassium, Calcium, Zinc, Iron, Riboflavin
Collard Greens, Cooked	A, C, K, B6 Folate, Magnesium, Phosphorus, Potassium, Calcium, Zinc
Green Beans	A, C, K, Folate, Thiamine, Niacin, Calcium, Iron, Magnesium, Phosphorus, Potassium, Zinc
Brussel Sprouts	A, K, C, Magnesium, Iron, Calcium, Folate, Potassium, Manganese

Vitamin and Minerals Breakdown:

- Vitamin A: Essential for eye health, skin, and immune function

- Vitamin C: An antioxidant that supports immune function and skin health
- Vitamin K: Crucial for blood clotting and bone health
- Folate: Important for cell growth and development
- Calcium: Essential for strong bones and teeth
- Potassium: Supports heart health and blood pressure regulation
- Magnesium: Plays a role in muscle function and bone health
- Iron: A good source of iron, which helps carry oxygen throughout the body
- Phosphorus: Essential for bone health and energy metabolism
- Manganese: An antioxidant that supports enzyme function

Here are some of the numerous benefits you may experience as a result of consuming greens and cruciferous non starchy vegetables:

1. Help to regulate blood sugar levels.

2. Improves blood circulation in the body.

3. Supports bone health.

4. Helps with high blood pressure readings (hypertension)

5. Prevents anemia.

6. Supports brain health (improved cognition).

7. Increase in nitric oxide, which is great for heart health.

3. **Herbs**

Herbs have been used for centuries for their medicinal and health-promoting properties. This is why herbal tea, herbal drinks, or consuming herbs is a daily requirement during The Perfect 10.

Herbal Teas For Health

- Ginger Tea - May improve headaches and blood sugar levels.
- Chamomile Tea - May improve anxiety, premenstrual cycle symptoms, acne, and sleep.
- Peppermint Tea - May improve nausea, upset stomach, and allergies.
- Hibiscus Tea - May help reduce blood pressure and improve cholesterol levels.
- Lemon Tea - May help with digestion. May boost immune system.
- Dandelion Root Tea - May be good for liver health, May help prevent urinary tract infections
- Green Tea - May decrease cognitive decline as you age. May improve heart health.
- Wild Burdock Tea - May work as a decongestant.
- Cilantro - May assist in removing heavy metals from the body.

Many of these herbs are also found in the "L.E.T.S. Health Perfect 10 Detox Tea."

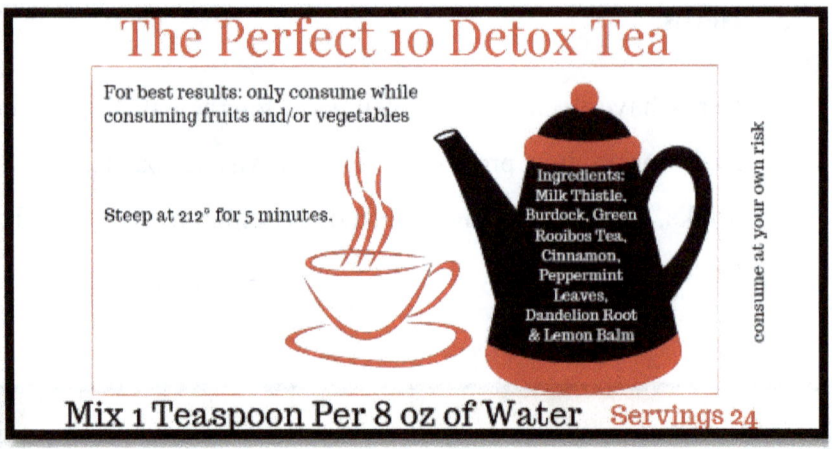

4. **Low Fat**

High-water-content fruits, botanical fruits, and non-starchy vegetables are all low-fat foods. These foods assist the pathway-elimination process by providing vital nutrients to the body and keeping it properly hydrated.

No oils of any kind are allowed. Oils are 100% fat. The Perfect 10 program focuses on low-fat plant foods and no added fats to those plant foods.

Whether a person purposely overeats fat or overtly overeats it due to it being found in plant food, the bottom line is too much fats cause weight loss to be at a standstill. Too much fat in the diet will cause weight gain, especially when consuming a high carbohydrate diet.

I'm not making fat be the bad guy. However, overconsumption of fat, especially trans-fat and saturated fat, has been linked to obesity, clogged arteries, blood flow issues, high cholesterol, stroke, heart attack, cancer, and even type 2 diabetes.

5. **High Fiber**

High water content fruits, botanical fruits, and non-starchy vegetables are all high-fiber foods. These foods assist the pathways elimination process by providing vital nutrients.

Fiber not only helps with weight loss. Fiber also helps you feel full, prevents constipation, helps keep blood sugar levels under control, and helps keep the digestive tract healthy by clearing out harmful waste.

Here are some great examples:

Juicy Fruits	**~Fiber In Grams Per 1 cup**
Grapes	1-2
Cucumber	1
Tomato	2-3

Apples	2-3
Blueberry	3-4
Strawberries	3-4
Raspberries	8
Pineapple	2
Mandarin Orange	2

Non-Starchy Vegetables	~Fiber In Grams Per 2 Cups
Asparagus	3.6
Broccoli	4.8
Romaine Lettuce	2.6
Green Cabbage	5.6
Cauliflower	5
Spinach	1.4
Kale	2.6
Collard Greens	10.6
Green Beans	5.4
Brussel Sprouts	6.6

6. No Added Sugars, Oils, or Salt (No SOS)

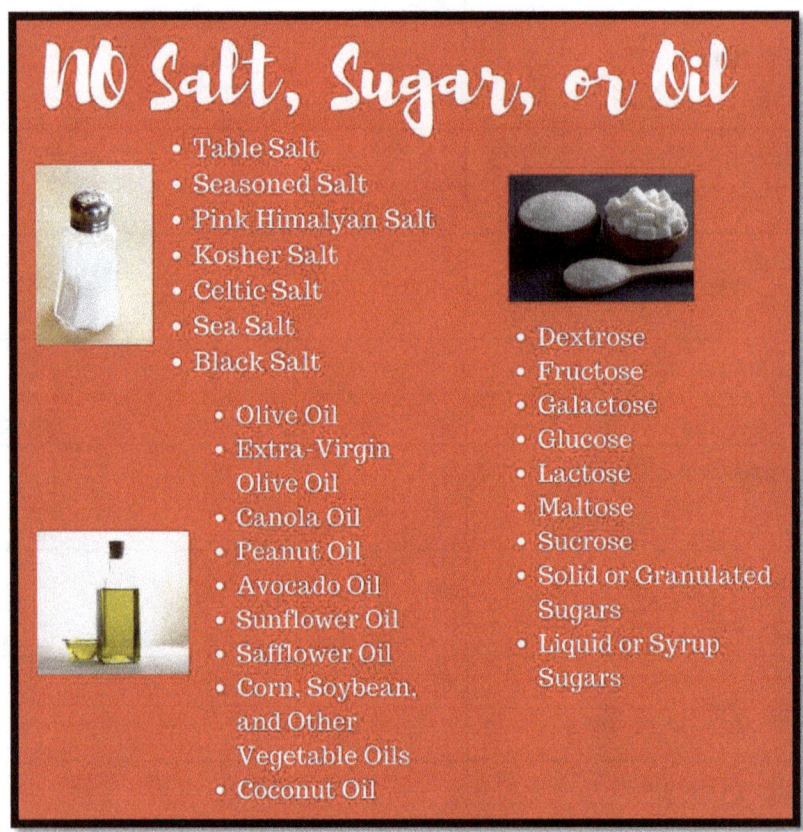

Sugars, oils, and salt are the main ingredients in processed foods for a reason. They are cheap, addictive, and give an immediate dopamine high. However, the cons outweigh any "good tasting" pros. Sugar, oils, salt, "SOS", consumption can lead to heart disease, diabetes, hypertension, dementia, stroke, cancers, and unfortunately the list of ailments goes on.

Excess sugar is converted into fat which leads to obesity. Excess sugar also leads to inflammation in the body. For instance, inflammation in the stomach is known as gastritis. Inflammation in the joints is known as arthritis and inflammation in the lungs is known as bronchitis. Sugar has also been linked to cognitive decline and dementia, and Alzheimer's have been referred to as "type 3 diabetes" as it closely resembles type 2 diabetes risk factors.

7. Proper Hydration

Hydration can be achieved in two ways, by what we drink and by what we ingest. Drinking water is a great way to hydrate the body and so is eating juicy fruits (as juicy fruits have a high water content).

Water is extremely important to our overall health. Water helps carry oxygen to the cells in the body. Without water, we would die. Water makes up more than 70% of our body. It makes everything flow.

Also, the more you sweat, urinate, and release fluids from your body, the more you need to stay on top of your hydration (and increase the amount you take in, to replenish what you lost).

8. Sea Vegetables

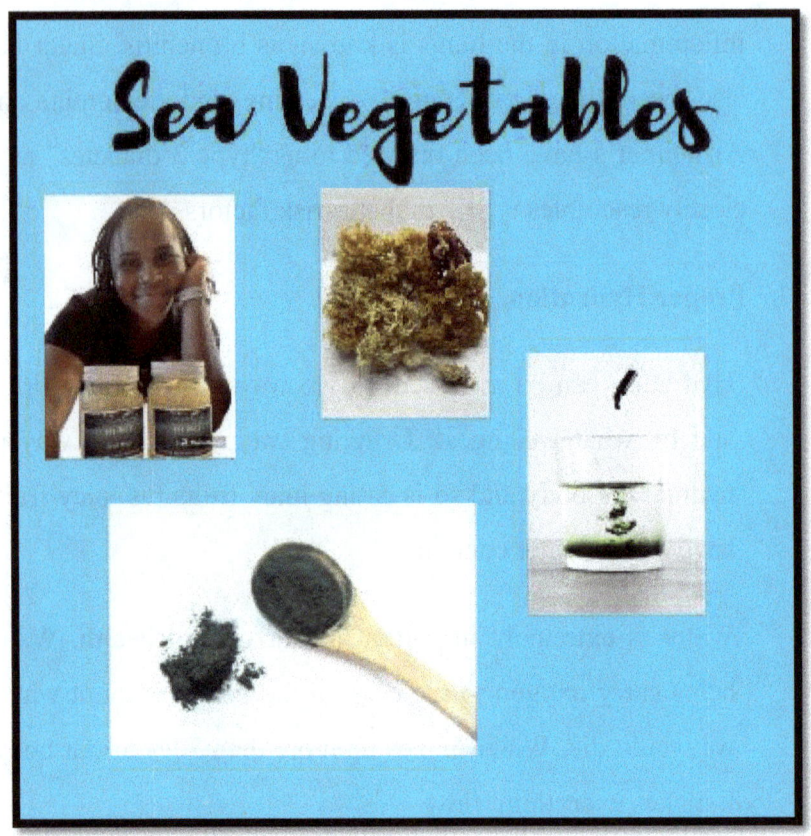

Sea vegetables include sea moss, bladderwrack, spirulina, chlorella, and kelp.

Sea moss is mostly found in the Caribbean but can also be located in various bodies of water around the world.

1. Sea moss contains about 92 of the 102 minerals found in the human body.

2. It may help support the body's immune system, respiratory system, and heart health.
3. It may also help improve skin, hair, energy, sexual health, and thyroid health.
4. May improve high cholesterol and hypertension.

Bladderwrack is an edible brown seaweed.

1. It may aid in weight loss.
2. It may help with eliminating joint pain, and urinary tract infections.
3. It is rich in fiber, antioxidants, and Vitamin B12, and may help relieve constipation.
4. May reduce inflammation.

Spirulina is a blue-green algae found in both fresh water and salt water.

1. May improve muscular strength and endurance by increasing the amount of time it takes before a person becomes tired.
2. A great source of protein, as it contains about 4 grams of protein per serving.
3. May help reduce high blood pressure.
4. May lower LDL, the bad cholesterol, and triglyceride levels and increase HDL, the good cholesterol, levels.

Chlorella is a green algae found in freshwater.

1. May protect against dementia.

2. May boost the immune system.

3. Because of its Vitamin B12 properties, it may help boost brain power. Also, if you follow a plant-based diet, B12 is a necessary supplement to your diet.

4. May help get rid of the body of toxins such as mercury.

Kelp is a type of seaweed that is brown and grows in saltwater.

1. Great source of iodine, calcium, iron, magnesium, folate, and Vitamin A.

2. May help increase energy levels.

3. May help boost brain function.

4. Supports brain health.

9a. Movement

1. Walking, cycling, and the elliptical are great steady-state cardio options.

2. At a minimum, walking and stretching should be done daily. Other forms of exercise are also encouraged based on your current exercise level.

3. HITT-style workouts are a great way to achieve fat loss. HIIT stands for "High Intensity Interval Training". The difference between steady cardio and weight training is that HITT training is when there are short bursts of intense exercise alternated with low-intensity recovery. For example, 30 seconds of jumping jacks followed by 15 seconds of walking in place. Then repeat those same high bursts of energy and low-intensity recovery for a specified amount of time.

9b. Sleep

The American Academy of Sleep Medicine and Sleep Research Society, adults aged 18-60 need at least 7 or more hours of sleep each night. Sleeping less than 7 hours per night regularly is associated with adverse health outcomes, including weight gain and obesity, diabetes, hypertension, heart disease and stroke, depression, and increased risk of death.

https://aasm.org/resources/pdf/pressroom/adult-sleep-duration-consensus.pdf

As your body detoxifies, you may feel fatigued or have the urge to lie down. Please listen to your body and rest as necessary.

10. Digestion Times

Fruit (and most veggies) are perfect for this as the digestion times are short. The Perfect 10 makes sure that an abundance of fruits and specific vegetables are consumed. This schedule of eating ensures the body is not in a state of constant digestion. That way the body can focus on the cleansing (removal) process of backed-up processed foods, junk foods, meat, etc. versus always digesting.

Both processes rely heavily on the fact that our bodies can either digest foods or cleanse them. It can't do both simultaneously. Because of this fact, cleanses tend to rely on easy and fast-digesting foods. That way your body can have time to eliminate toxins.

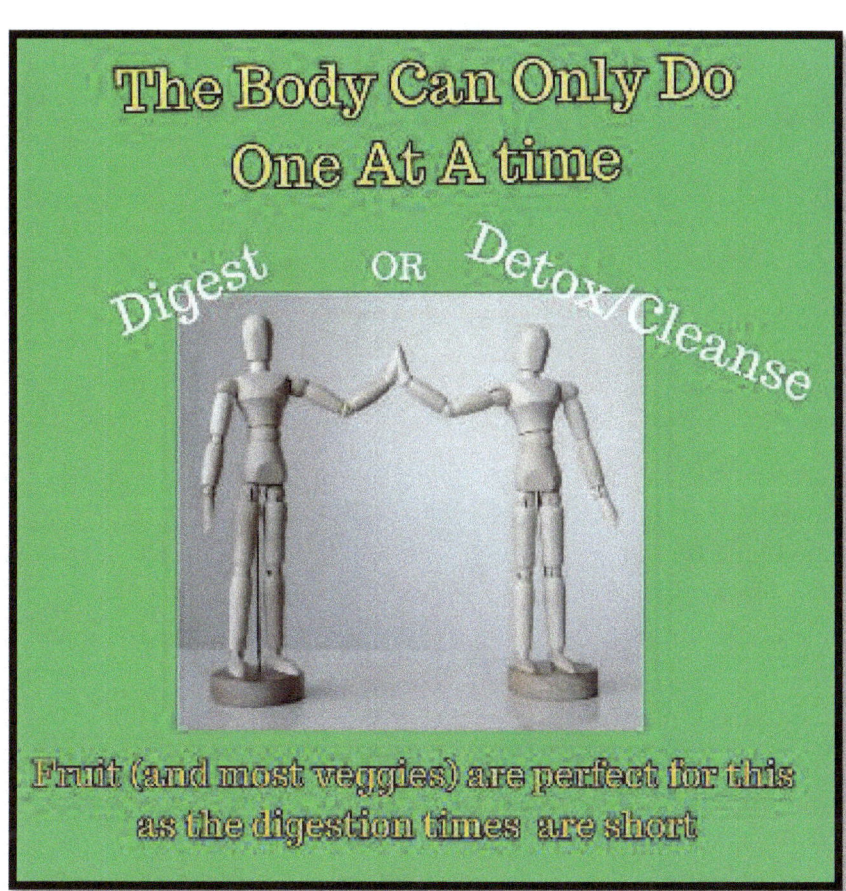

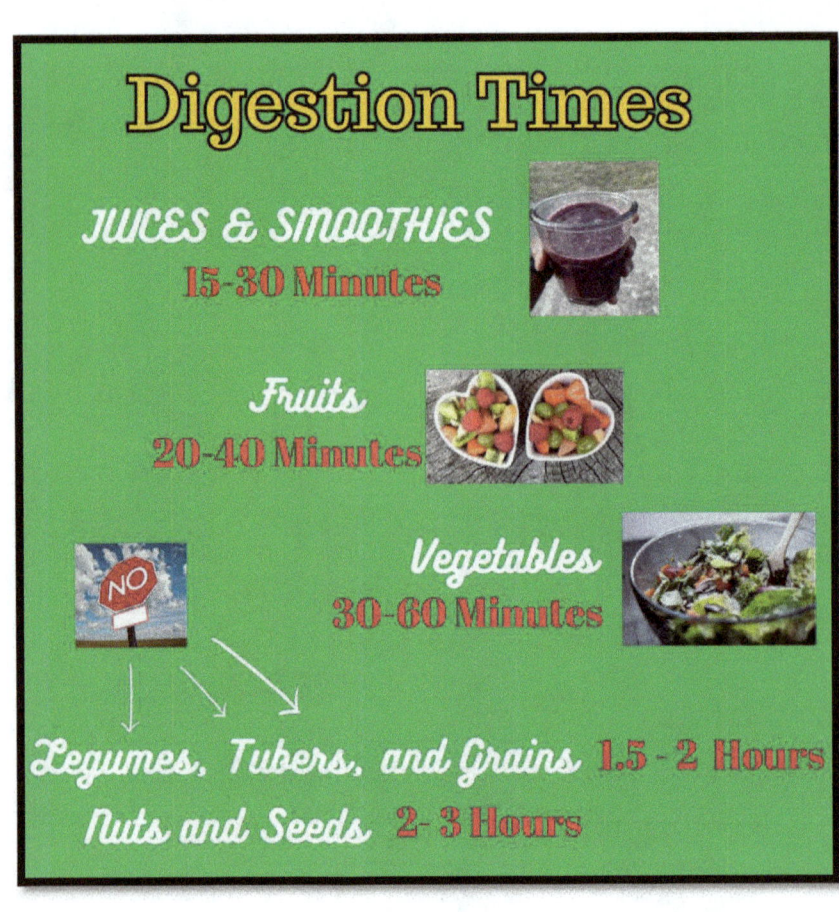

The Perfect 10 Detox gradually increases in nutritional difficulty as you progress from one phase to the next. For example, the first 5 days (Phase 1) will allow the option of cooked veggies, whereas the next 3 days (Phase 2) will not allow any cooked veggies, only raw vegetables and fruits, and then finally, the last 2 days (Phase 3) will be fruits only.

Gradually increasing the difficulty will allow your body to adjust more gently to the changes in your diet. There will still be detox symptoms for most, but the severity of them will depend on what diet you are coming from. If you are coming from a heavily processed or fatty/sugary/salty diet, then you may have more detox symptoms than someone who is coming from a more whole foods-based diet.

The Perfect 10 Detox is a 3-phase program that will follow a "yes list", "no list", and phase-specific guidelines.

Take your time and review this list, this will help you stay on track as well as answer common questions about what you can consume.

YES LIST

1. High Water Content Fruits
2. Non-Starchy Vegetables
3. Herbs
4. Botanical Fruits
5. Hydration
6. Herbal Tea
7. Sea Vegetables
8. Movement/Sleep
9. Approved Condiments, Sauces, Broths
10. Caffeine (no more than 50 mg per day if needed)

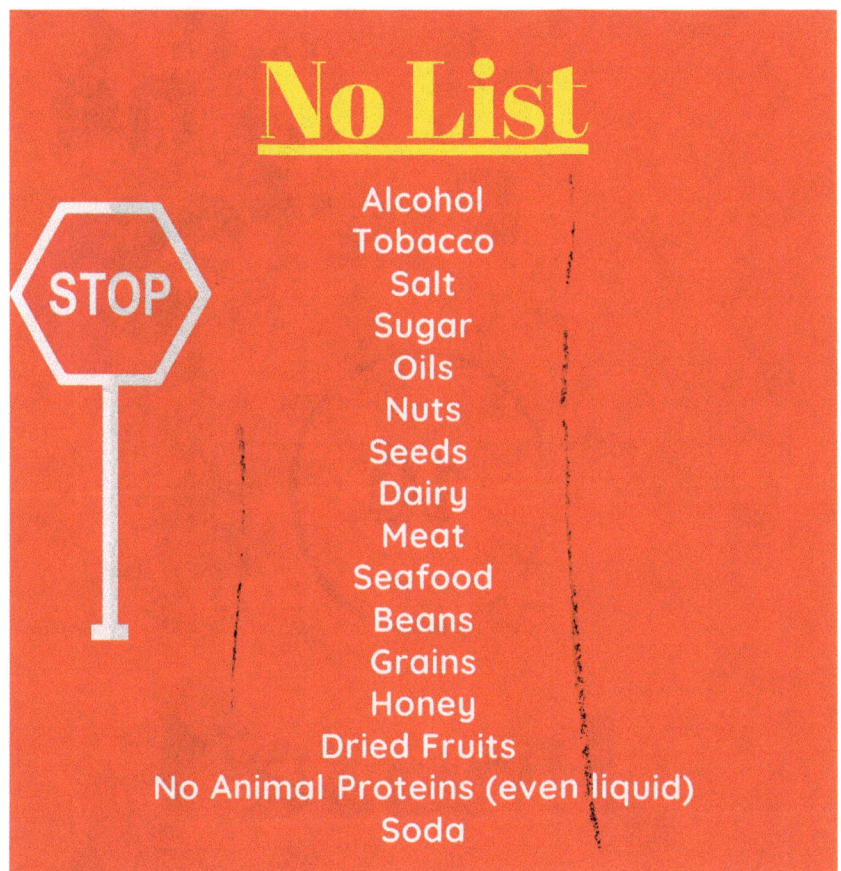

Each phase breakdown will include:

1. The Rules
2. Fruits/Botanical Fruits Grocery List
3. Non-Starchy Vegetables Grocery List
4. Herbs List
5. Sample Daily Plan

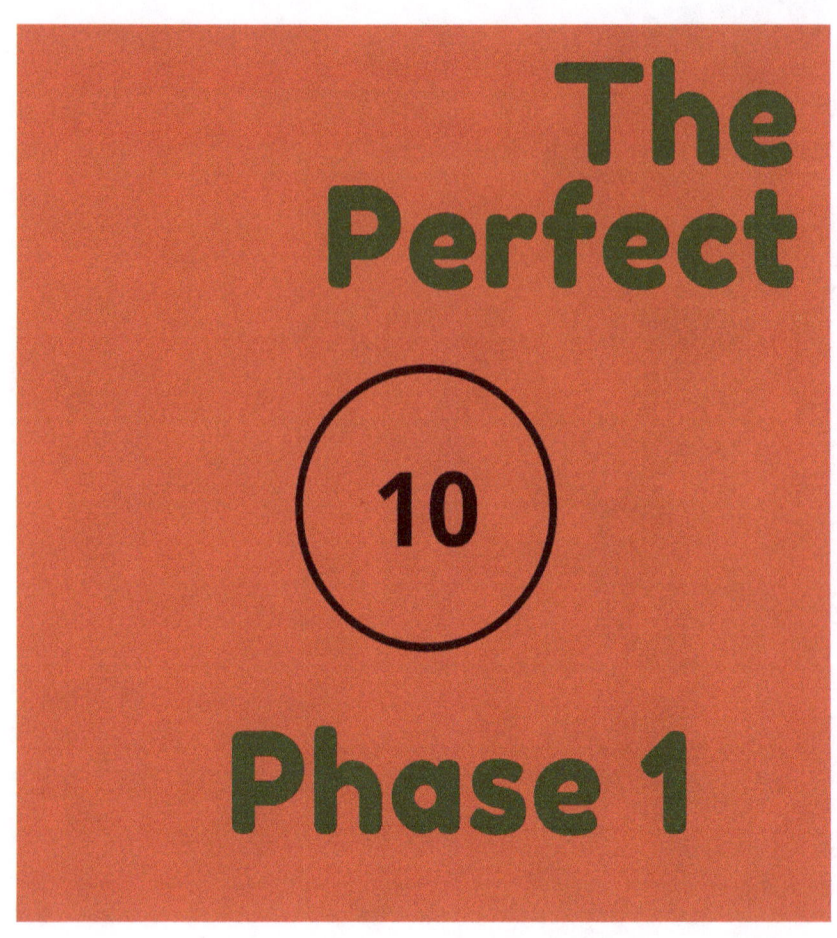

Chapter 5

The Perfect 10 Phase 1

Phase 1 is the first 5 days of the cleanse. During the first five days, both raw and cooked fruits and vegetables can be consumed. The only legume that is allowed is chickpeas (which is technically a fruit as well).

You can elect to only eat fruit during phase 1 instead of the designed program. You can also elect to only consume your fruits and vegetables raw during phase 1. Those are the only modifications you can make.

The detox rules are built around the "Yes and No List", but with some specific guidelines for Phase 1.

Phase 1
The Rules

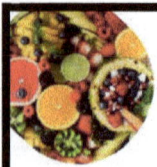

Day 1-5

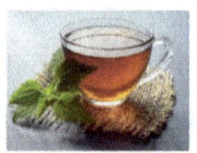

- All juicy fruits allowed
- All non-starchy vegetables
- All botanical fruits
- Fruits and veggies can be consumed raw or cooked
- Cooking methods include: baked, air fried, juiced, microwaved, or boiled
- No oils allowed
- Drink herbs everyday
- Cooked chickpeas allowed
- 1-2 bananas per day are allowed
- No dates allowed
- No avocado
- No olives
- 1/4 cup grape nuts per day or something similar (optional)

The grocery list below is not all-inclusive, which means there are other non-starchy vegetables and fruits that you may consume. However, my recommendation is that you stick to this list as much as possible as these tend to be high water content non-starchy vegetables, botanical fruits, and fruits.

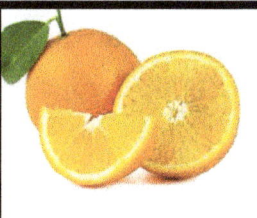

Grocery List – Phase 1
Raw or Cooked
All Juicy Fruits Allowed

JUICY FRUITS
- Grapes
- Grapefruit
- Strawberry
- Blueberry
- Blackberry
- Raspberry
- Mangoes
- Watermelon
- Cantaloupe
- Apples
- Pears
- Kiwi
- Persimmons
- Nectarines

JUICY FRUITS
- Rambutan
- Lychees
- Soursop
- Banana (see Phase rules)
- Papaya
- Passion Fruit
- Guava
- Pineapple
- Lime
- Lemon
- Oranges
- Mandarins
- Plums
- Peaches
- Cherries

Eat them, Blend them, or Juice them

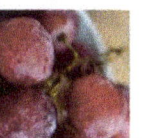

Grocery List – Phase 1
Raw or Cooked
Non-Starchy Vegetables

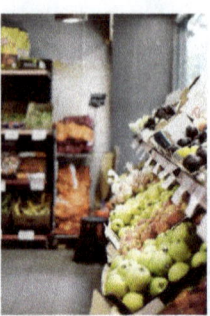

Tip: only buy what you actually enjoy eating

Artichoke
Asparagus
Bean Sprouts
Beets
Brussels Sprouts
Broccoli
Cabbage (green, bok choy, purple)
Cauliflower
Celery
Greens (collard, kale, mustard, turnip)
Hearts of Palm
Leeks
Garlic
Mushrooms
Okra
Onions
Pea Pods
Peppers
Radishes
Salad Greens (chicory, endive, escarole, lettuce, romaine, spinach, arugula, radicchio, watercress)
Sugar Snap Peas
Swiss Chard
Turnips
Water Chestnut

Grocery List – Phase 1
Raw or Cooked
Botanical Fruits and Extras

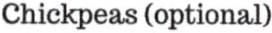

Tip: only buy what you actually enjoy eating

Chickpeas (optional)
Banana (no more than 2 per day)
Grape Nuts Cereal (optional, no more than 1/4 cup per day)
Bell Peppers
Peppers - any kind
Cucumber
Zucchini
Tomato
Pumpkin
Squash - any
Eggplant

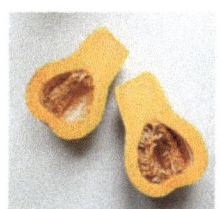
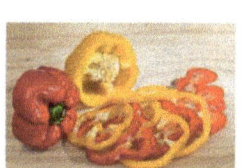

Grocery List
Phase 1
HERBS

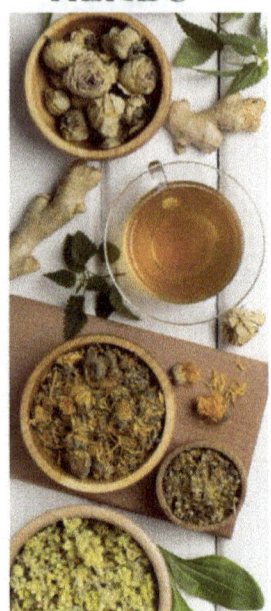

Herbal Tea
Ginger Tea
Chamomile Tea
Peppermint Tea
Hibiscus Tea
Lemon Tea
Dandelion Root Tea
Green Tea
Wild Burdock Tea
Soursop Leaves Tea
Sorrel Tea

Herbs
Basil
Cilantro
Dill
Mint
Oregano
Parsley (Italian)
Parsley (Curly)
Rosemary
Milk Thistle

You may be wondering about dressings and sauces. This graphic shows you what dressings, marinades, and sauces you can and cannot have. If you can go without condiments, do that. If you do choose to use condiments, use only what's necessary.

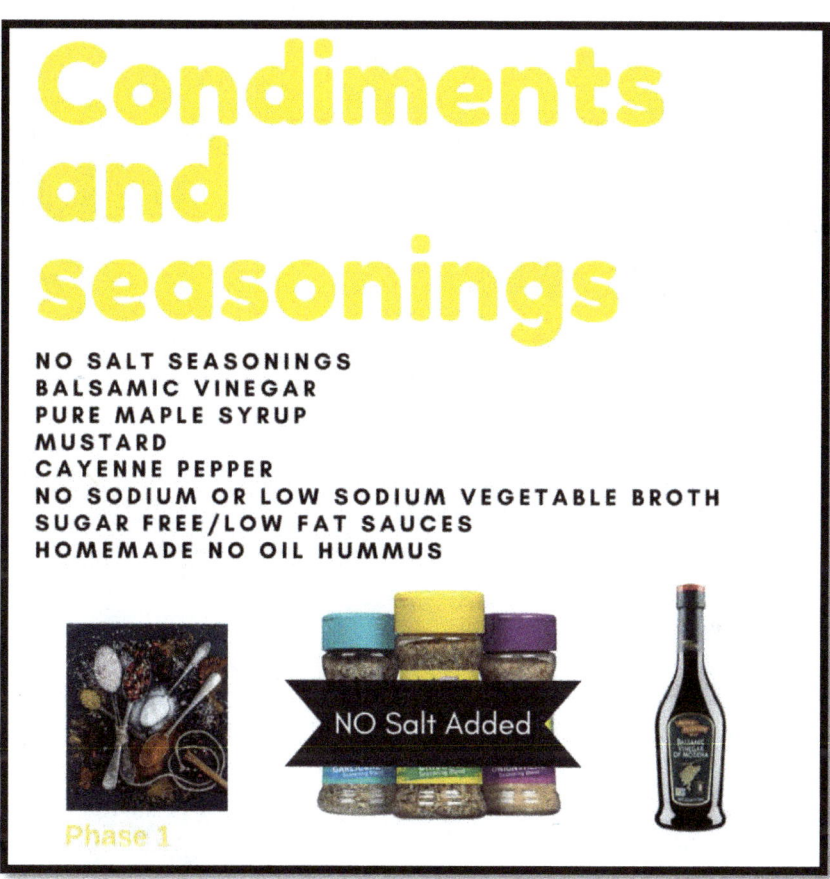

My suggested plan for phase 1 is outlined in the graphic below. This plan focuses on consuming your herbal tea or herbal drink first thing in the morning with a veggie stir fry or smoothie, eating cooked veggies throughout the day, snacking on fruit, and then finishing your day with some more cooked vegetables, chickpeas, or even cooked squashed makes for a fulfilling day.

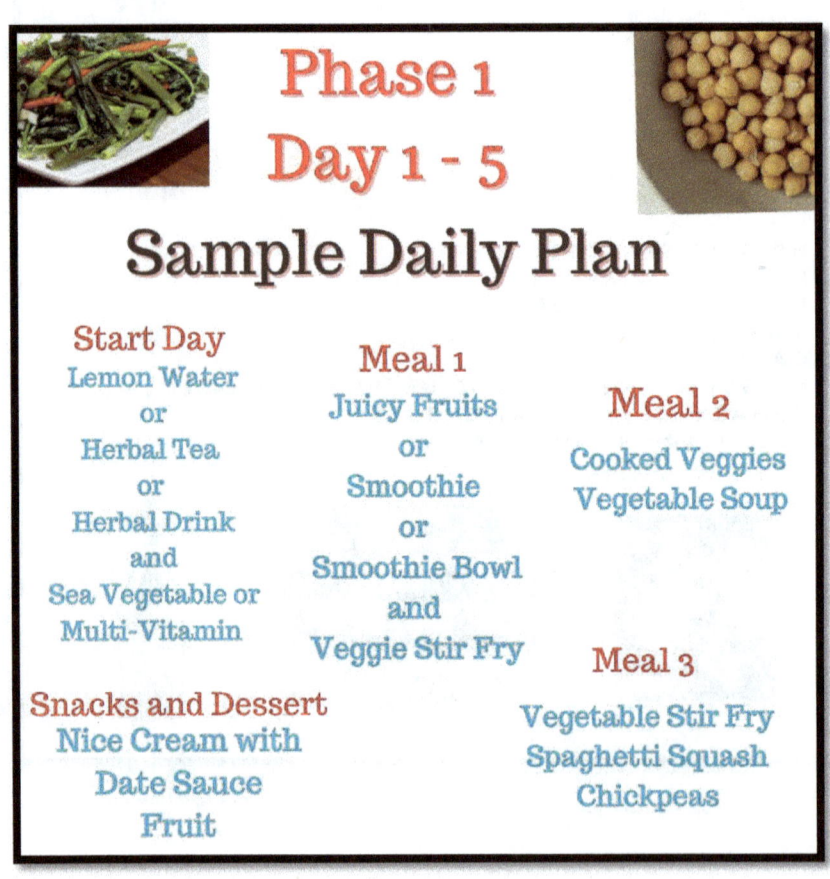

Phase 1
Day 1 - 5

Sample Daily Plan

Start Day
Lemon Water
or
Herbal Tea
or
Herbal Drink
and
Sea Vegetable or
Multi-Vitamin

Meal 1
Juicy Fruits
or
Smoothie
or
Smoothie Bowl
and
Veggie Stir Fry

Meal 2
Cooked Veggies
Vegetable Soup

Meal 3
Vegetable Stir Fry
Spaghetti Squash
Chickpeas

Snacks and Dessert
Nice Cream with
Date Sauce
Fruit

Preparation for your cooked fruits and vegetables is very specific. You must use the following methods of preparing fruits and vegetables:

- Air Fryer – foods prepared in the air fryer are typically marinaded, seasoned, and then air-fried.

- Pan Fry – only use water, broth, balsamic vinegar, or some other "no oil" based liquid in preparation of vegetable preparation. Feel free to add minced garlic, diced onions with the liquid of choice. This will create a flavorful base for the stir fry.

- Boil- vegetables like carrots, cabbage, and collard greens, tend to stir fry easier and are easier to chew once boiled first.

- Microwave- place vegetables into a microwave safe dish, add a little water or broth (and seasoning), then microwave.

- Bake – Similar to an air fryer, add seasoning to the vegetables then put in oven safe dish/pan and bake.

- Grill – foods can be marinaded and seasoned before applying to a grill.

- Juice – use a juicer to process fresh fruits and non-starchy vegetables.

- Smoothies – use a blender to combine your favorite fruits and/or vegetables, add water, fresh, juice or coconut water as your base, and blend.

- Smoothie Bowls- use bananas, acai or other blended frozen fruit as the base. Then top with the desired fruits.

Remember: You cannot use oil to prepare your food. Use water or low-sodium (no sodium) vegetable broths instead.

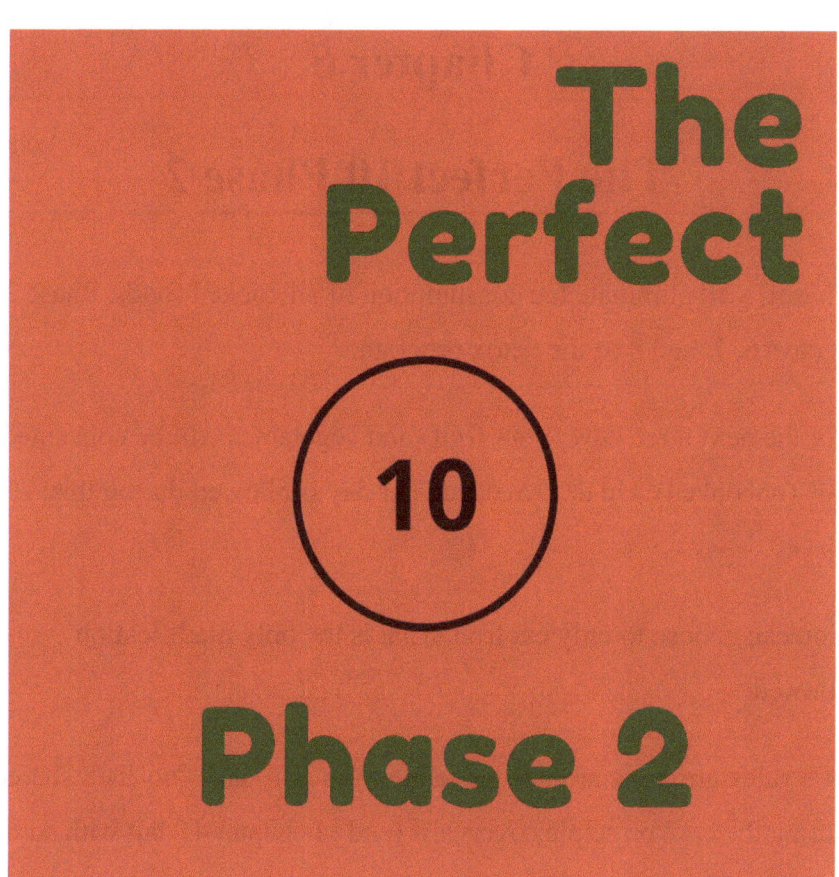

Chapter 6

The Perfect 10 Phase 2

Phase 2 will eliminate the consumption of all cooked foods. Phase 2 is days 6, 7, and 8 of the detox program.

For the next three days, your fruits and vegetables will be consumed raw (uncooked). Up to ½ avocado per day is allowed during this phase.

You can choose to only eat fruit. That is the only modification allowed.

The rules are built around the same "yes list" and "no list" shared during the core principles overview (end of chapter 4), but with some specific guidelines for Phase 2.

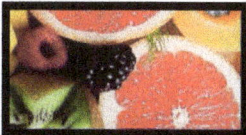

Phase 2
The Rules

Day 6, 7, and 8

- All food must be consumed RAW
- All juicy fruits
- All non-starchy vegetables
- All botanical fruits
- No oils
- No dehydrated foods
- Drink herbs everyday
- 1-2 Bananas per day
- 1-3 Dates allowed per day
- 1-5 Olives allowed per day
- 1/2 Avocado allowed per day
- Cooked exception: homemade chickpea hummus allowed

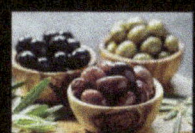
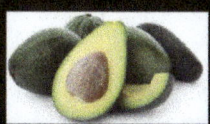

The grocery list for phase 2 is not all-inclusive, which means there are other non-starchy vegetables and fruits that you may want to consume. My recommendation is that you stick to this list as much as possible as these tend to be high water content non-starchy vegetables, botanical fruits, and fruits.

If you would like another type of fruit that's not listed, do a basic internet search, "water content of xxx fruit". If it has 80% or higher water content, and zero fat, then you can consume it.

Grocery List – Phase 2
All Raw
Non-Starchy Vegetables

Tip: Only buy what you actually enjoy eating

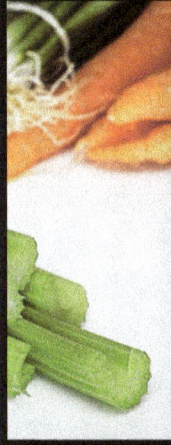
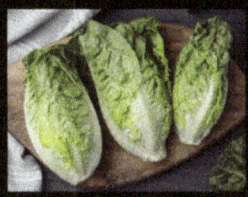

Mushrooms
Onions
Radishes
Salad Greens (chicory, endive, escarole, lettuce, romaine, spinach, arugula, radicchio, watercress)
Sprouts
Zucchini
Beets
Celery
Greens (collard, kale, mustard, turnip)
Swiss Chard
Hearts of Palm
Leeks
Carrots

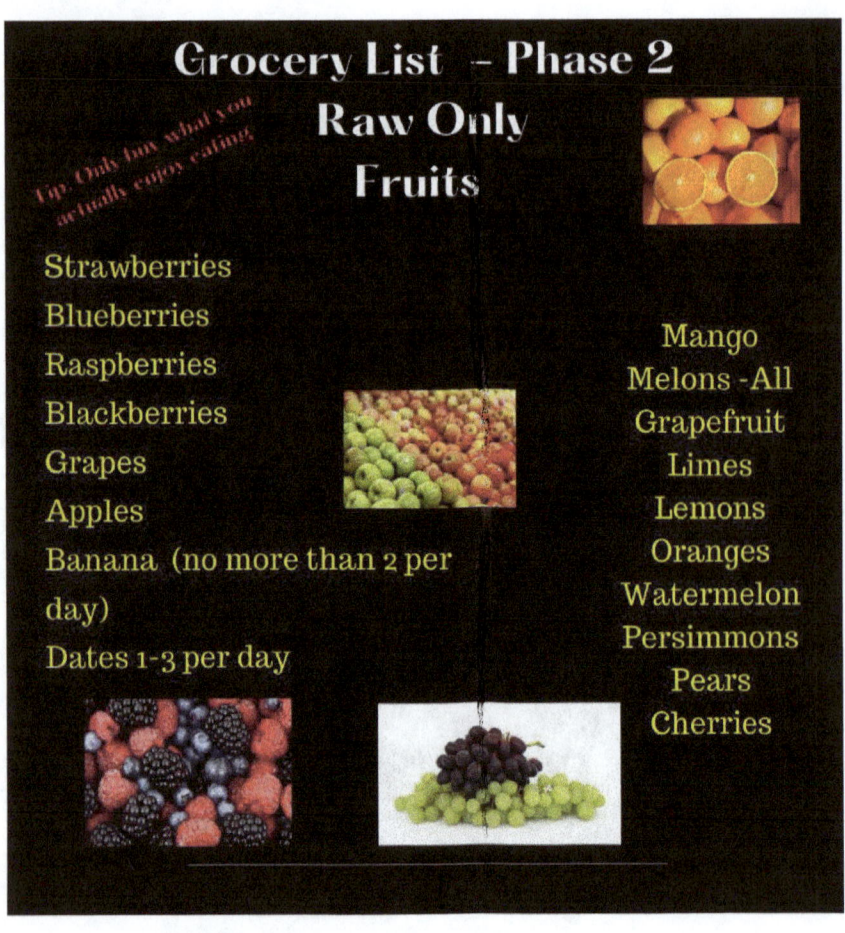

Grocery List – Phase 2
Raw Only Fruits

Tip: Only buy what you actually enjoy eating!

- Strawberries
- Blueberries
- Raspberries
- Blackberries
- Grapes
- Apples
- Banana (no more than 2 per day)
- Dates 1-3 per day
- Mango
- Melons - All
- Grapefruit
- Limes
- Lemons
- Oranges
- Watermelon
- Persimmons
- Pears
- Cherries

Preparation methods for your raw fruits and raw vegetables are very simple. You can simply just eat the fruits and vegetables as is, or you can "prep them" if you choose.

- Mono Eat- this is where you only eat one fruit per sitting (meal), or one fruit for the entire day.

- Fruit Salads – combine fruits with salad greens or by themselves. You can also top with blended fruit as a "dressing".

- Juice – using a juicer, or blender (with strainer), juice desired fruits, herbs, and vegetables and drink them.

- Smoothies – using a blender, blend desired fruits, herbs, and vegetables and drink them.

- Smoothie Bowls – using a blender or food processor, use bananas, acai or other blended frozen fruit as the base. Then top with the desired fruits and toppings.

- Salads – combine non-starchy vegetables with fruit and/or herbs. Eat as is, or top with an approved condiment, sauce, or dressing.

- Wraps – use collards, kale, or even romaine as wraps, load them up with your favorite fruits or vegetables, and approved sauces, and eat them like a taco or burrito.

- Veggie Platters – take your favorite veggies, arrange on a platter, and enjoy with vegetable-based dips or on their own.

Phase 2 dressings and sauces will have to be prepared by using balsamic vinegar, mustard, maple syrup, avocado, fruits, and vegetables. Avocado can be added to wraps, and platters, as well as used to create salad dressings. It is very versatile.

You cannot use oils.

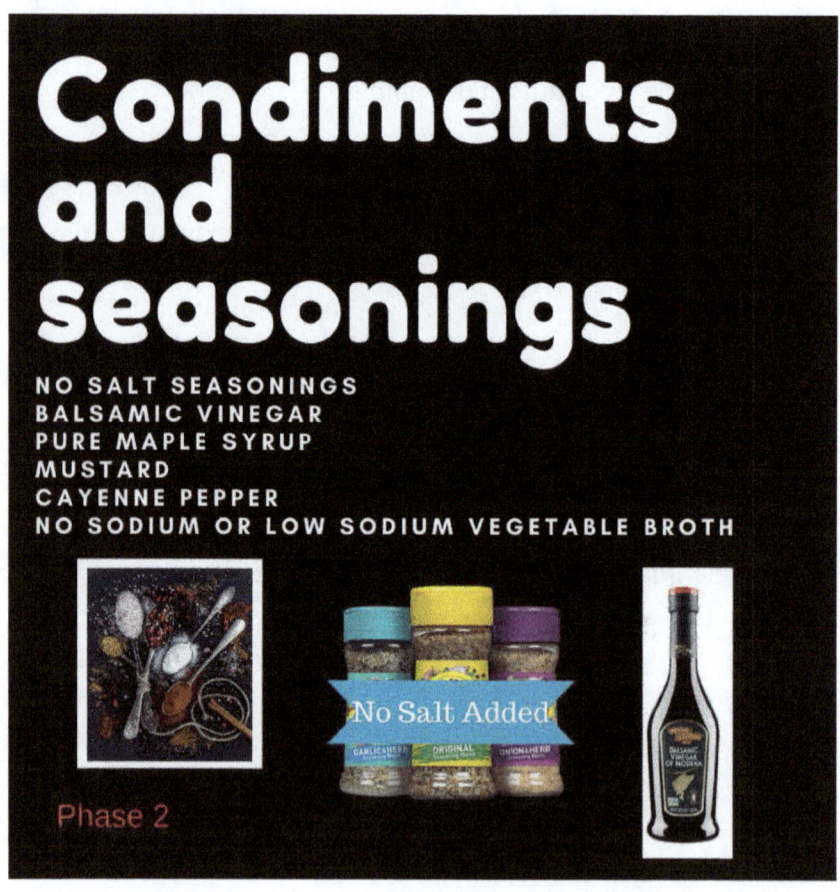

My sample daily eating plan for phase 2 is outlined in the graphic below:

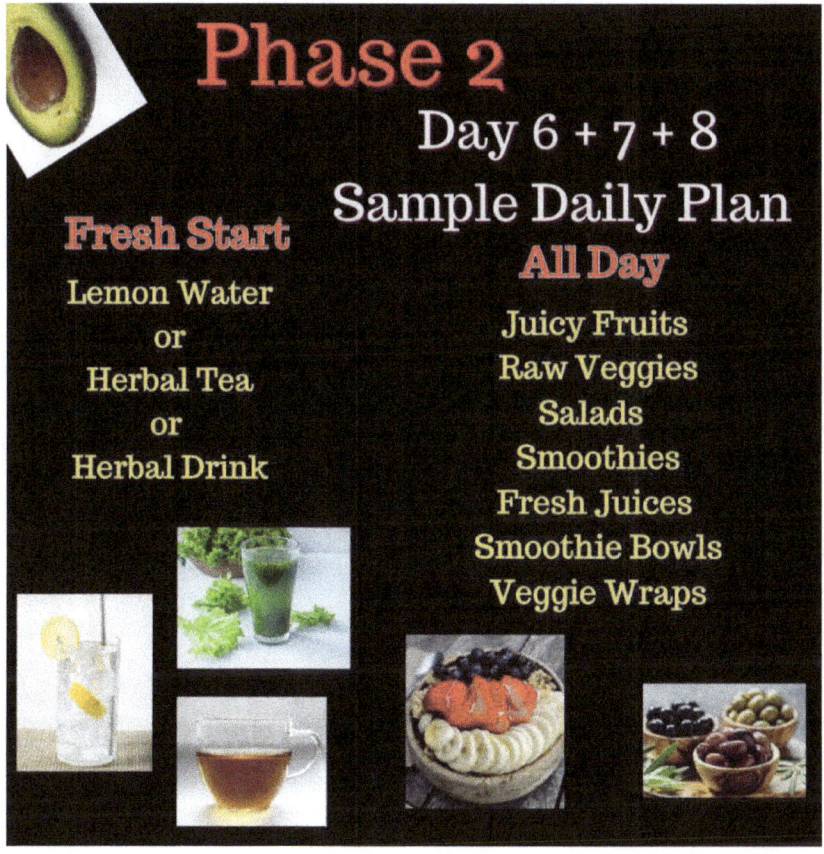

Remember this is merely a sample suggested day. You do not have to follow this outline.

The Perfect

(10)

Phase 3

Chapter 7

The Perfect 10 Phase 3

Phase 3 is days 9 and 10 of the detox.

Phase 3 will remove the consumption of all vegetables. For the next two days, fruits (both traditional and botanical fruits) will be the only plant foods you can consume.

Beets will be the only exception to this rule, raw juiced beets, are allowed to be consumed during phase 3.

The rules for phase 3 are built around the "no list", but with some specific guidelines for phase 3.

Take a look below:

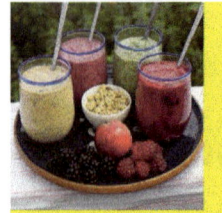
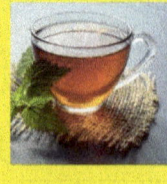

Day 9, 10
Phase 3
The Rules

- All juicy fruits allowed
- All botanical fruits allowed
- Drink herbs everyday
- No dehydrated foods
- No more than 2 bananas allowed per day
- 1-5 Dates allowed per day
- No olives
- No avocado
- Beets allowed (must be raw)

My suggested sample plan for phase 3 is simple. CONSUME FRUIT. There is no timetable for when you can or cannot consume fruit. You can blend it, juice it, or just eat it. Up to you. Below I've included an idea of how you may want to arrange your day.

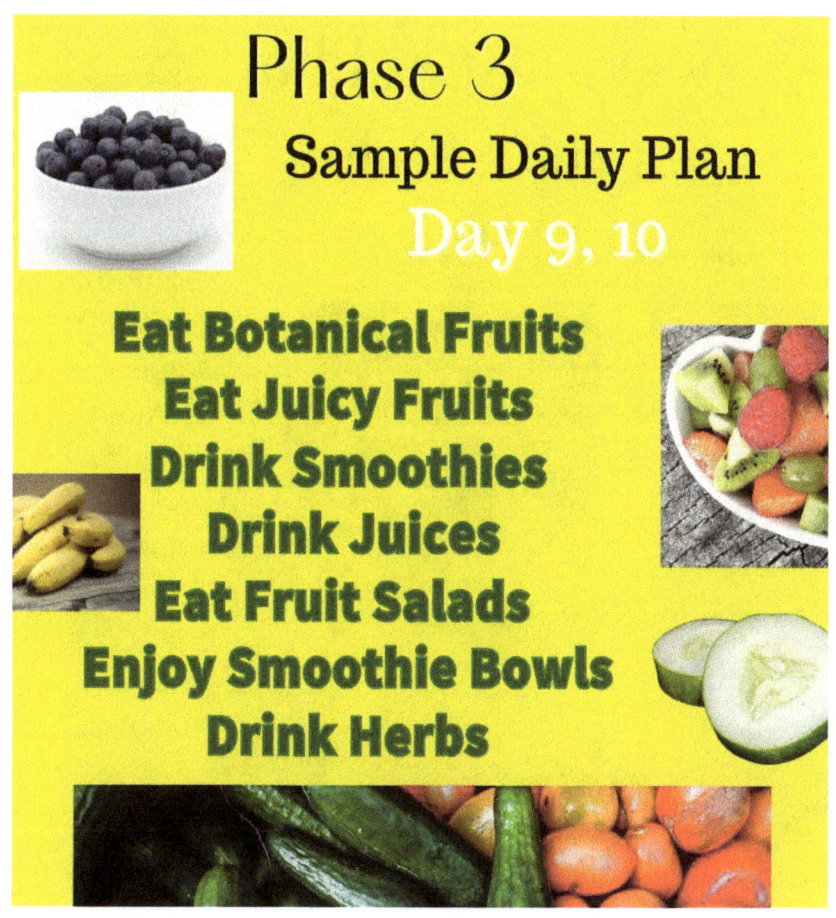

The grocery list below is not all inclusive of fruits that you may consume. The only non-fruit allowed during this phase is beets.

Grocery List – Phase 3
Fruits Only
All Raw

Tip: Only buy what you actually enjoy eating

Strawberries
Blueberries
Raspberries
Blackberries
Grapes
Apples
Cherries
Banana (no more than 2 per day)
Dates (no more than 5 per day)

Oranges
Mango
Melons-All
Grapefruit
Limes
Lemons
Persimmons
Dragon Fruit
Pears
Coconut Water
Kiwi
Pineapple

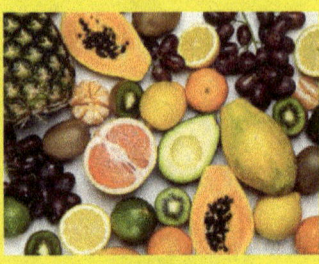
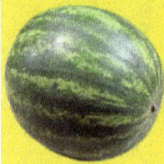 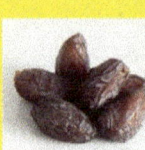 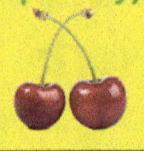 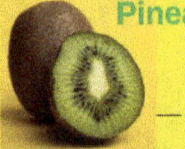

Grocery List – Phase 3
All Raw
Botanical Fruits and Extras

Ginger
Turmeric
Herbal Tea - Any
Basil
Cilantro
Dill
Mint
Oregano
Parsley
Rosemary

Tip: Only buy what you actually enjoy eating

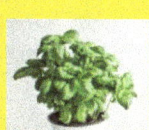

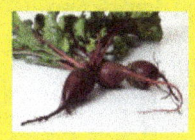

Bell Peppers
Peppers - Any kind
Cucumber
Zucchini
Tomato
Yellow Squash

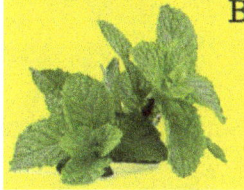

Beets (must be raw)

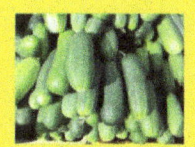

Preparation for your raw fruits is very simple. You can just eat fruits as is or you can "prep them".

Here are some ideas below for raw fruit preparation:

What about dressings/sauces during phase 3? Balsamic vinegar and pure maple syrup are the only dressings/sauces allowed.

- Mono Eat- only eat one fruit per sitting (meal), or one fruit per day.

- Fruit Salads - combine fruits, then top with lemon or lime juice.

- Juice- juice desired fruits and drink them.

- Smoothies - blend desired fruits and drink them.

- Smoothie Bowls – use bananas, acai, or other blended frozen fruit as the base. Then top with the desired fruits.

Condiments and seasonings

NO SALT SEASONINGS
BALSAMIC VINEGAR
PURE MAPLE SYRUP
MUSTARD
CAYENNE PEPPER

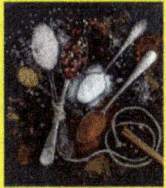
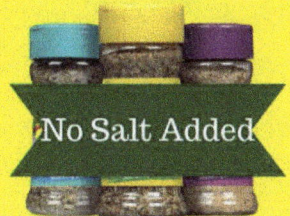
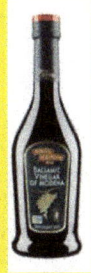

Phase 3

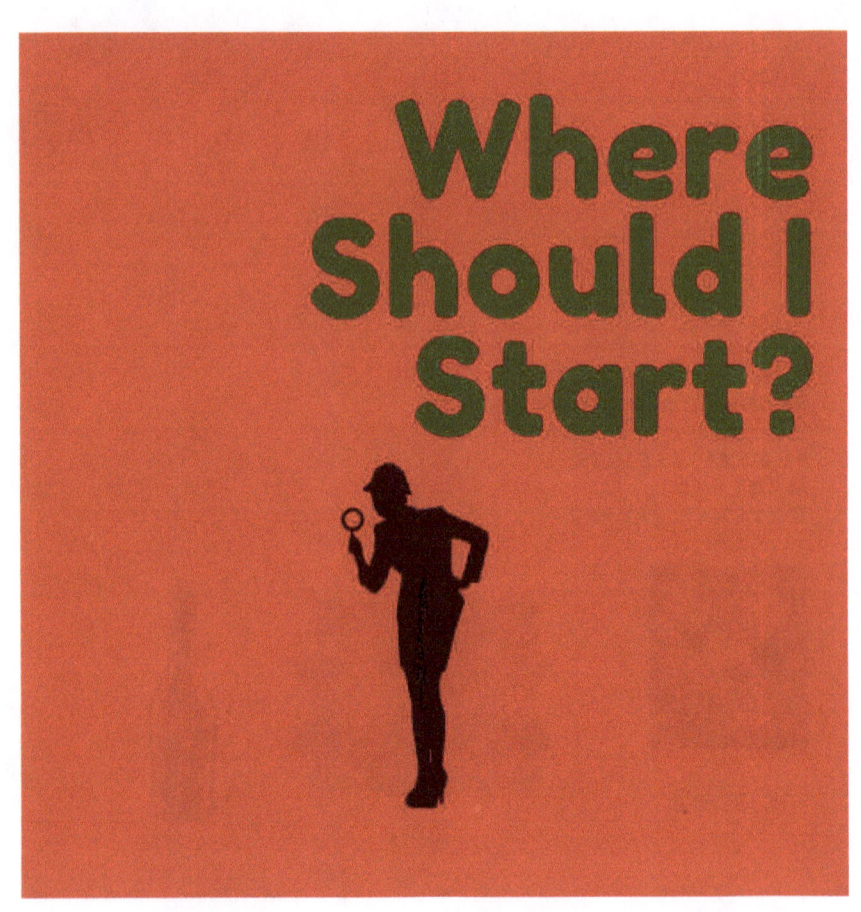

Chapter 8

Where Should I Start?

My suggestion is to follow the Perfect 10 Detox program from phase 1 to phase 3. However, I do recognize that everyone comes from different backgrounds, experiences, and levels of cleansing (and healthy eating) and may want to start in stay in phase 1, 2, or 3 because of that. Your current health, weight, or needs may also influence what phase you would like to start with. Because of these reasons, I have outlined some program modifications and levels to meet everyone where they are.

Level 1 Detoxer (Beginner)

If you are a beginning-level "detoxer", or someone who would like to progressively go through a detox with a "gentler" approach, then starting with level 1 would be ideal.

A level 1 detoxer may also be a person who has not completed a detox/cleanse program before, may have not completed a detox/cleanse program in a long time, or tends to eat an unhealthy diet regularly.

If level 1 is your starting point, then I suggest you follow The Perfect 10 program from phase 1 through phase 3 over 10 days.

Phase 1 = 5 Days in length

Phase 2 = 3 Days in length

Phase 3 = 2 Days in length

Some participants may prefer to stay at phase 1 for the whole 10 days. Phase 1 tends to be a gentler detox experience. Great results will still occur if this option is chosen.

Level 2 Detoxer (Intermediate)

If you are a more experienced "detoxer", this means you fast from time to time, routinely complete a cleanse, or eat clean daily, then you could choose to begin The Perfect 10 starting from phase 2 and progressing to phase 3. You could double the time spent in phase 2 (6 days), and double the time spent in phase 3 (4 days) for a total detox time of 10 days.

Phase 2 = 6 Days in length

Phase 3 = 4 Days in length

Some participants may prefer to stay at phase 2 for the whole 10 days. Phase 2, although more challenging than phase 1, tends to be a gentler detox experience than phase 3. Great results will still occur if this option is chosen.

Level 3 Detoxer (Advanced)

If you are an advanced level "detoxer", this means you routinely detox or fast, as well as eat super clean. More advanced detoxers, may choose to start at phase 3 of the Perfect 10 Deteox. If this option is chosen, a time frame of 3-10 days would be in phase 3.

$$\text{Phase } 3 = 10 \text{ Days}$$

Some participants may prefer to only complete phase 3. Phase 3 can be completed for a period of 3-10 days. Phase 3 tends to be the most challenging of all the phases.

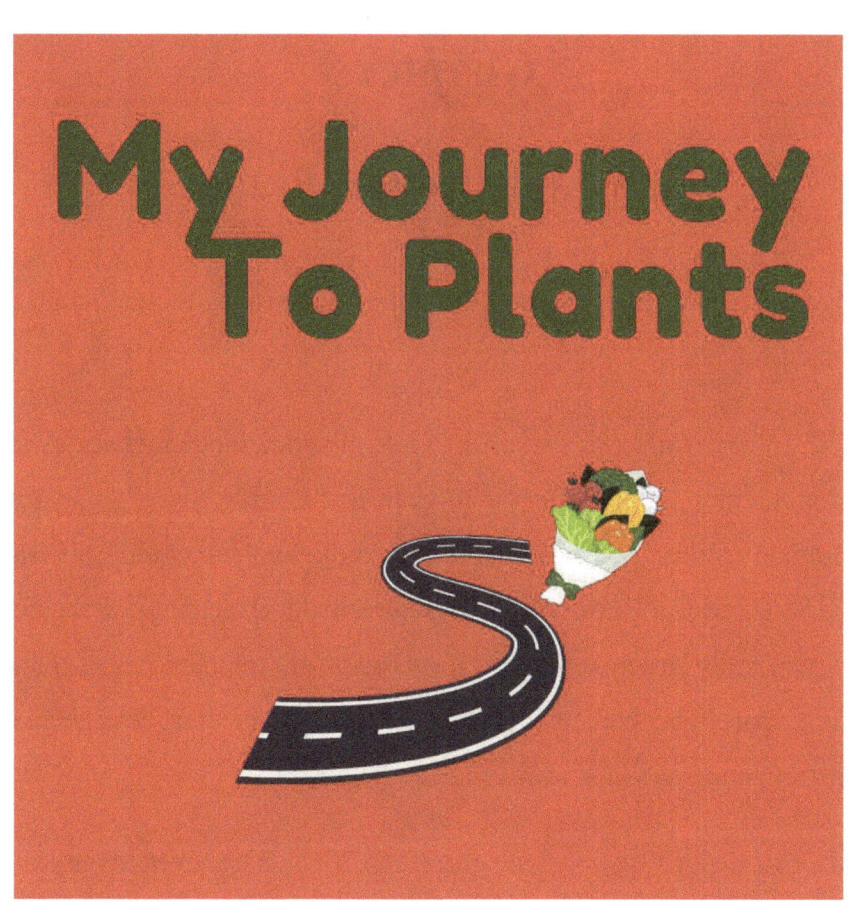

Chapter 9

My Journey to Plants

I've had a few major personal situations that proved to me that plant results are real!

In 2015, my world was shaken up. First, my grandmother passed away from kidney failure after a 20-year battle with type 2 diabetes, multiple strokes, seizures, inability to walk, and dementia. This was the hardest death I've ever had to endure, and it changed the dynamics of our family structure forever. It was also very traumatizing, as I had been a part of her care team and witnessed those medical emergencies from a young age (and always felt so helpless).

The first major situation that occurred in 2015, that proved to me plant results are real, was that I was diagnosed with pre-diabetes and was overweight. To some that may not seem like such an impactful situation, but after what I witnessed my grandmother suffer through, the diabetic diagnosis felt like a death wish. And worse, my physician at the time offered no solutions, he just told me that when the time came, he would prescribe medication.

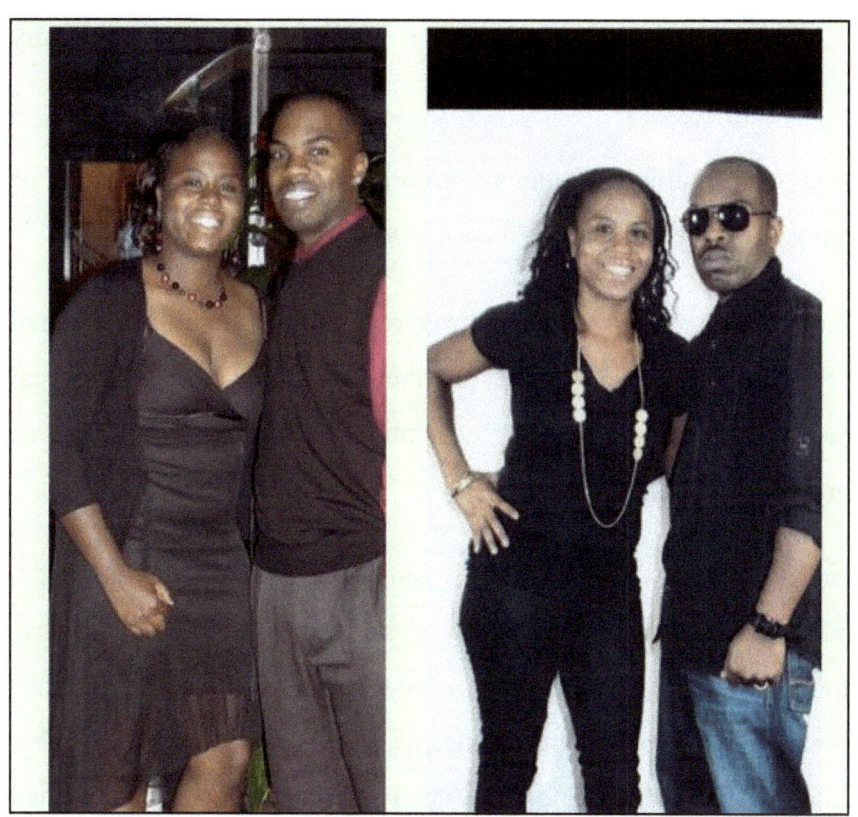

Although this news was devastating, it led me down a path of using plant foods to heal. I was determined not to follow in my grandmother's footsteps and have my quality of life impacted. This is how I first discovered plant-based results. I implemented a whole food, plant-based plan and reversed the diabetes. I felt 10 years younger and lost more than 20 pounds in the process. I was hooked on feeling amazing.

RESULTS DON'T LIE!

I'd like to say that's the only time that "plants came to the rescue" and saved my life, but it wasn't.

Friday, April 22, 2022. My life forever changed. This would be my 2nd major situation.

What seemed like it would be a normal day turned into a day of emergency and ultimately a day of God's grace.

That morning, I dropped off my two daughters to school and headed to Starbucks, grabbed a coffee, and then went to my job as a physical education and health teacher at a middle school. All of that was normal.

Once at work, I went through my first few classes feeling "normal", and then around lunchtime, things began to feel weird. And by weird, I mean my body started feeling out of sorts and doing things it didn't normally do. The first occurrence was at lunch. I was eating and suddenly felt nauseous and threw up. Then shortly after lunch, we had a fire drill and while walking out to the evacuation site, I continued to feel strange, almost like I was out of my body. It was as if I was "floating", and my heart was beating so fast.

I attempted to finish my coffee, thinking maybe I was just tired and needed some caffeine. I took a Tylenol thinking maybe I was just coming down with something. But nothing made me feel better. I ended up leaving work mid-day still feeling, "out of body".

As I was driving home, I felt like my vision was in slow motion, my heart was racing, and I felt tightness on the left side of my neck and upper shoulder area. My bra also felt tight around my chest, like I was suffocating. As I reached out to family members, they kept asking me, "What's wrong? What do you feel?" I just could not seem to find the words to describe what I was feeling.

I just knew something was wrong. Something was off.

I thought to myself, am I having a stroke? Am I having a heart attack? Am I going to die?

Hours later I found myself at an urgent care center being evaluated for a possible heart attack, diabetic episode, and/or a stroke. Thankfully, I passed all the tests for low blood sugar and stroke symptoms. But they did discover my blood pressure was elevated, and my heart was still racing. They decided to give me an electrocardiogram (EKG).

After being told that my EKG was abnormal, my husband and I were told to go to the emergency room immediately. I was terrified! More terrified than I have ever been in my entire life. All I could think about was dying and leaving my daughters without a mother. Or going into the hospital, "normal", and coming out medically disabled.

I have seen close family members suffer from life-changing strokes and life-ending aneurysms, so the fear of going into the hospital as "Ange", and coming out disabled, or not coming out all, was real.

Once at the hospital, I was given another EKG. They also took blood work, and based on the findings of the EKG, I was taken into triage immediately. All the commotion and the body language of the ER medical staff was scary to observe. They were concerned that I was having a heart attack. I spent hours having my blood pressure and heart rate monitored via blood pressure cuff, and heart electrodes attached to my chest.

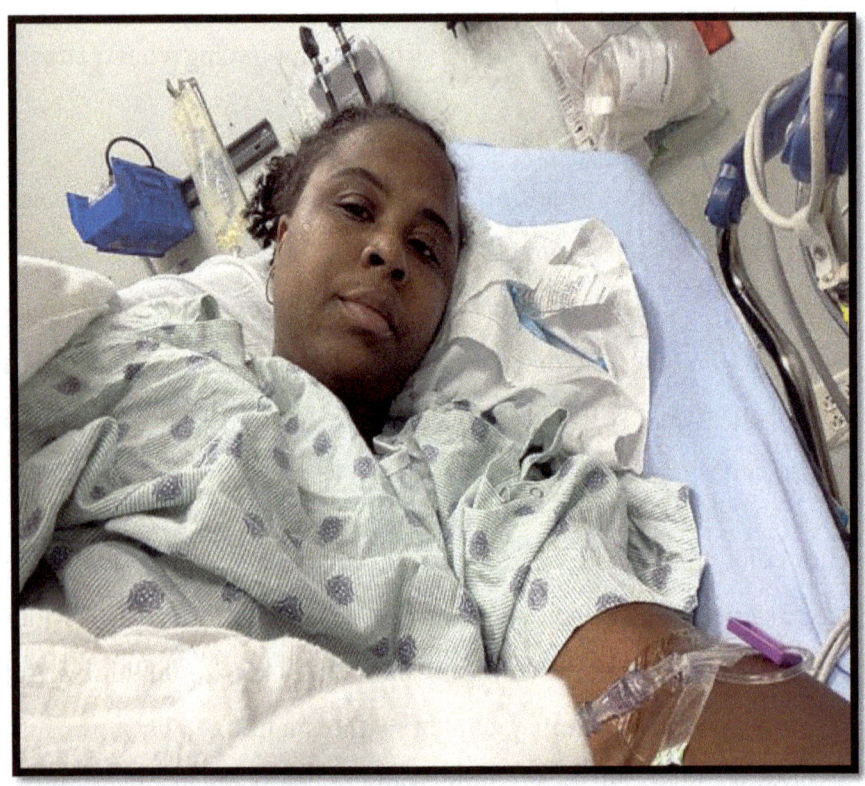

I was given the following diagnoses and a to-do list:

#1 I was pregnant! Yes, at age 38 (and without planning), I was pregnant. Based on that I was told that I needed to see an OB/GYN.

#2 Due to the abnormal EKG, I would need to see a cardiologist immediately. The emergency room did not have anyone on staff who could evaluate the readings for me, but based on the way the EKG results looked, they knew that my condition was serious.

#3 Due to the elevated blood pressure and rapid heart rate, I was told to see my primary doctor for a possible hypertension diagnosis.

Whew! I WAS OVERWHELMED! I was more worried about my health and well being than I had ever been in my life. I felt loss.

Now there were several issues with all of these "to dos", but one that intensified it all was this was a Friday night, and I would not be able to make calls to set up all these Doctor appointments by that Monday. This meant a weekend of unexplained high blood pressure, a weekend of worrying about what an abnormal EKG meant (exactly). Plus, a weekend of settling into the idea that at 38, I would be carrying my 3rd child (while trying to figure out what was wrong with my heart).

This caused a level of anxiety that I had never experienced before.

The following weeks led to a miscarriage, an official anxiety diagnosis, and the search for a cardiologist.

Once I was able to meet with a cardiologist, I was placed on Family Medical Leave Act (FMLA) from work until my heart issues were diagnosed, resolved, and I could safely return to full-time teaching.

After months of seeing and receiving care from my cardiologist, I experienced:
1. Multiple echocardiograms conducted.

2. Wearing a heart monitor for 24 hours a day for 3 weeks.
3. Having nuclear stress test (which felt like a simulated heart attack)
4. Logging my blood pressure twice a day then reviewing the logs with my cardiologist at our appointments (if you've never had to do this, it is nerve wrecking waiting to see what those numbers are).

Cardiologist diagnoses and recommendations:

It was determined that about 8 percent of my heart was not receiving oxygen. This in itself could lead to cardiac arrest or stroke.

To determine why only 8 percent of my heart was receiving oxygen, my cardiologist would need to go in to my body with a camera to look around the heart area (in question) and possibly conduct heart surgery while he was in there.

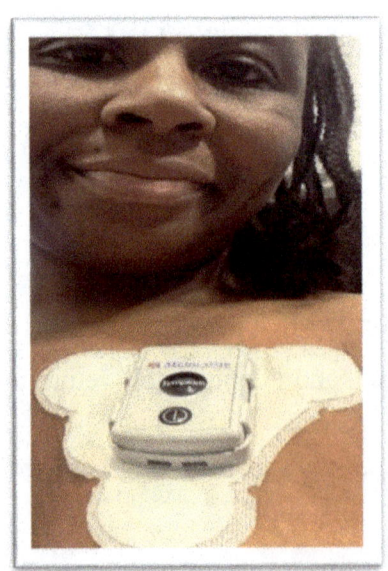

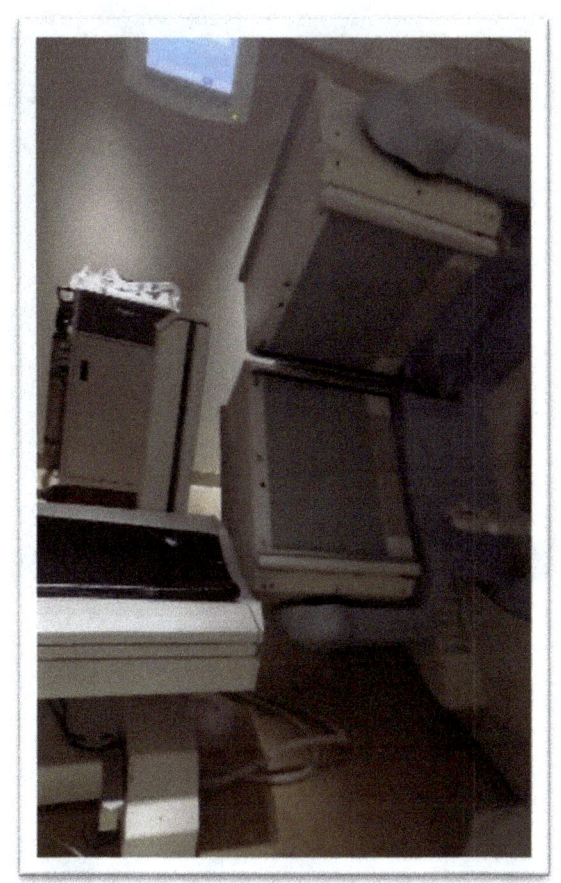

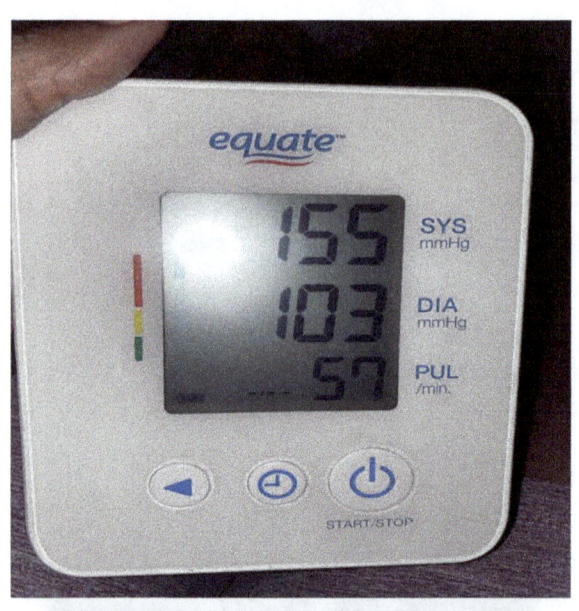
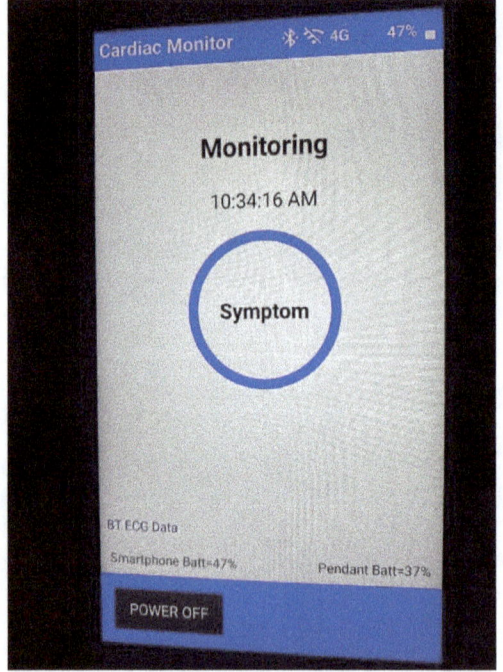

It was also suggested that I start hypertension medication to control the increased diastolic and systolic blood pressure readings.

During this "recommendation" appointment, I asked my cardiologist, "If I begin the medication to help me "maintain" normal blood pressure, will this be temporary or forever?" his reply was not the answer I was hoping for, he said, "Once you start, you will continue them forever".

I thought to myself, no way! I'll use them in an emergency, but long term, for my life, I did not want that.

The other big decision I needed to make was to have them go into my body to determine the cause of the oxygen loss, and the possibility of having heart surgery once they did. The risk, in my opinion, were not worth it. I did not want to have heart surgery. I would instead lean on a different method.

I decided to use plants! Only this time would be slightly different from the plan I used in 2015. I needed a stricter plan that would warrant immediate results. I needed a cleanse/detox program.

This is when the beginning core principles of The Perfect 10 were born.

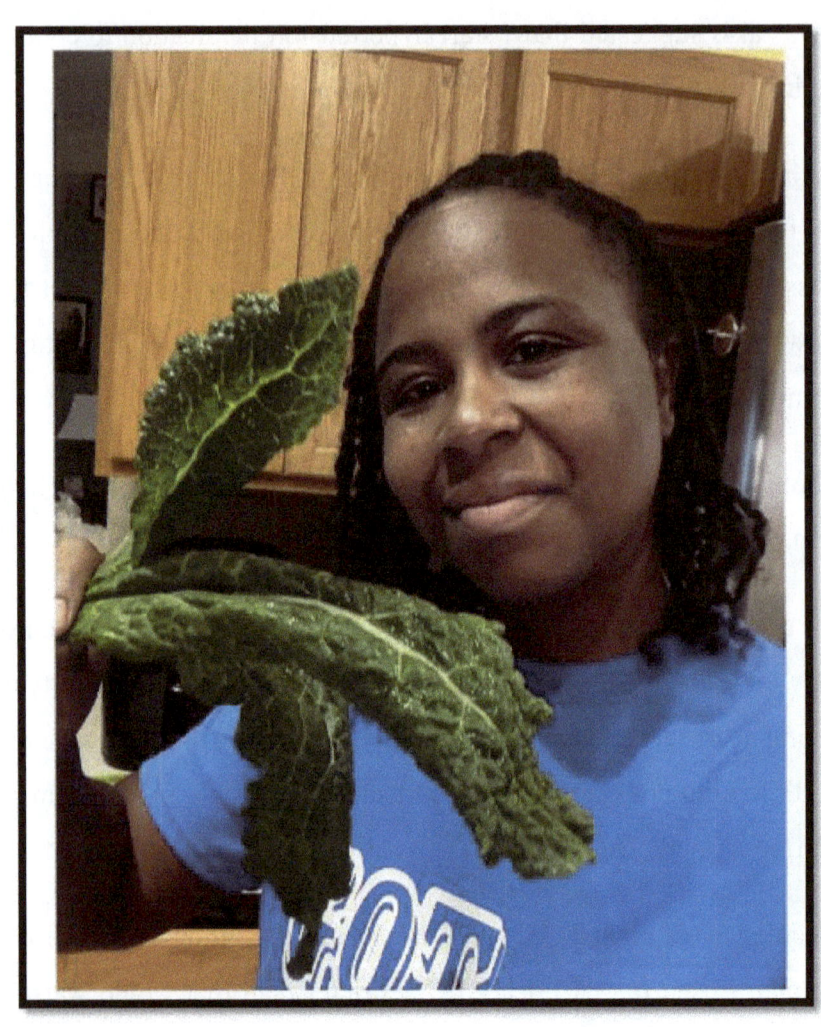

I immediately began implementing The Perfect 10 core principles. At every dr. appt after, I begin to see improvements in my blood pressure. My blood lab work showed increased HDL cholesterol (the good kind improved from 44 to 57) and lower LDL Cholesterol (the bad kind improved from 99 to 79), amongst other improved lab tests. My blood pressure was also normalizing! At my final diagnostic visit, the percentage of my heart not receiving oxygen had reduced as well, and I did not need hypertension medicine anymore. My cardiologist was shocked! He could not believe I had achieved all this without the help of medication or surgery. I told him I was just implementing good old-fashioned fruits and vegetables, exercise, and prayer into my daily plan.

RESULTS DON'T LIE!

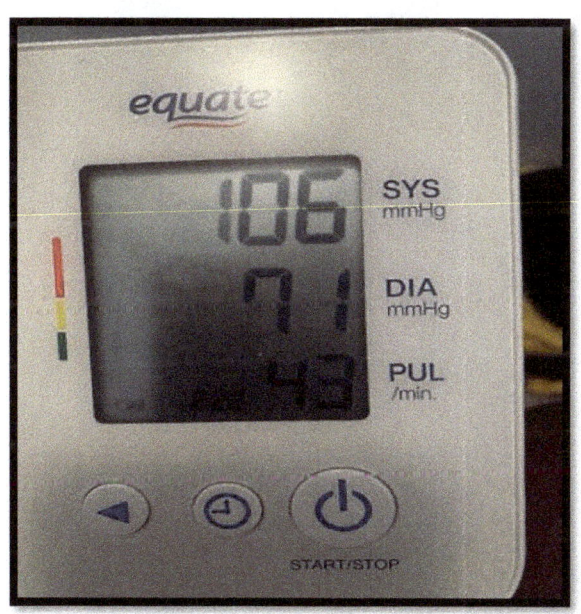

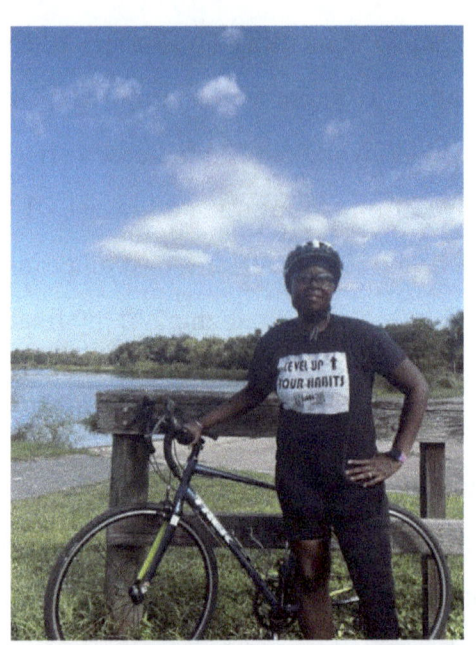

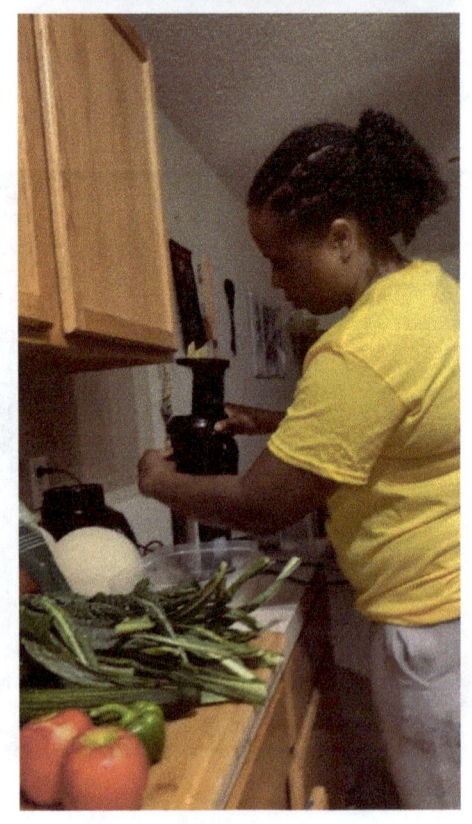

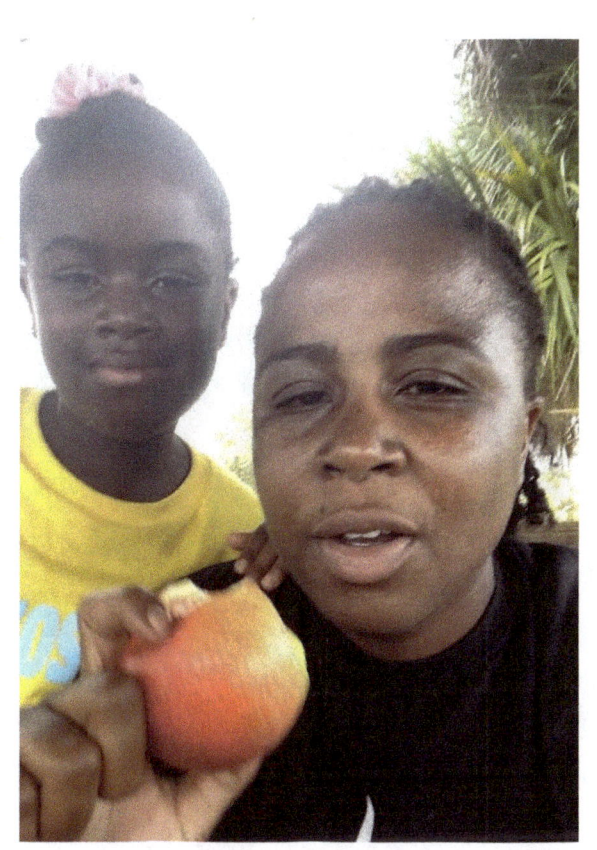

There Are No Dumb Questions

Chapter 10

There Are No Dumb Questions

After doing plant-based coaching for more than 8 years, working with a diverse group of individuals, and hosting detox groups, I've been blessed to come across the most common (and sometimes uncommon) questions.

Look through this list. The questions you may have, are likely answered here:

1. Why are we focusing on such a small list of fruits and vegetables?
2. Why can't I have grains, beans, nuts, or seeds?
3. What kind of water should I drink?
4. Can I use frozen fruits and vegetables?
5. Can I use canned vegetables?
6. What about diets that are high in fat, why are they successful with weight loss?
7. I am having cravings that I do not usually have. What might that mean?
8. How does increasing fiber help with chronic diseases?
9. How will I know if the detox is working?
10. What equipment do I need for The Perfect 10 Detox?
11. How do I best store fruits and vegetables so they stay fresh longer?

12. Will I lose belly fat?
13. Can I consume nut and seed butter (peanut butter, almond butter, etc.)?
14. Can I consume veggies that have been cooked with meat or animal broth?
15. What can I do if I am experiencing low energy?
16. Can I follow The Perfect 10 Detox long-term?
17. I do intense exercise, any pre-workout recommendations that aid with workout endurance and hydration?
18. Why do some of the recipes only have ingredients listed versus the measurements for how much to add?

1. **Why are we focusing on such a small list of fruits and vegetables?**

    Simplicity yields better results. When there is less to remember, it keeps the focus on healing.

2. **Why can't I have grains, beans, nuts, or seeds?**

    Nuts and seeds are high in fat. The Perfect 10 focuses on a low-fat diet cleanse. It is easy to overeat foods that are high in fat.

    Grains and beans have longer digestion times than fruits and vegetables. Remember the body can only do one of two things at a time, detox or digest. We want to focus on fast-digesting foods so that our bodies can use most of the time detoxing.

3. **What kind of water should I drink?**

    During the cleanse, drink distilled or spring water.

4. **Can I use frozen fruits and vegetables?**

   Yes! Frozen fruits and vegetables are a great option as they do not spoil or go bad as soon as fresh does. Frozen options are also typically less expensive than fresh fruit and vegetables.

5. **Can I use canned vegetables?**

   I'd suggest sticking to fresh or frozen. But if your budget or circumstance requires you to use canned vegetables then please read the ingredients. Before consuming any canned vegetables, read the food label. Specifically, you must read the ingredients. There should be no added salt, no added sugar, and no added fat. You can refer to the no list for guidance.

   If you are unable to find canned vegetables without added salt, rinse the vegetable thoroughly with water before consuming.

6. **What about diets that are high in fat, why are they successful with weight loss?**

   Well, high-fat diets usually have you cut carbs to achieve weight loss. We are not doing that! I am not here to argue for or against other dieting styles. Remember this book is about the power of plants and The Perfect 10 Detox. That's it. But I will say, that the overconsumption of fat, especially trans-fat and saturated fat, has been linked to obesity, clogged arteries, blood flow issues, high cholesterol, stroke, heart attack, cancer, and even type 2 diabetes. Fatty foods are not ideal for cleansing the body.

7. **I am having cravings that I do not usually have. What might that mean?**

    As mentioned before, sometimes the detox process comes with unwanted symptoms and cravings.

    5 major food cravings that most people experience are salty, sweets, chocolate, dairy, and red meat.

    Some cravings throughout the detox will be because of habit or a mental battle you will have to overcome. But true cravings are usually because the body lacks nutrients. Salty cravings could be a lack of trace minerals. Sweet cravings could be a lack of chromium. Chocolate cravings could be a lack of magnesium. Dairy cravings could be a lack of essential fatty acids. Red meat cravings could be a lack of iron and/or Vitamin B12.

    Use that information to fill in your diet with the missing nutrients to decrease those cravings.

8. **How does increasing fiber help with chronic diseases?**

    Fiber attacks chronic diseases in many of the same ways. I want to provide two quick examples (there are many more):

    Person A has high cholesterol.

    How would consuming fiber-rich foods help this person? Fiber is not absorbed in the intestine. It acts as a binder in our body and grabs ahold of cholesterol and fats and then releases them into our body's bloodstream. From there, cholesterol and fats can be released through defecation.

Person B has Type 2 Diabetes.

How does consuming foods rich in fiber help this person? Our body cannot break down fiber into glucose like it does other carbohydrates. The body also cannot absorb fiber. Because of these two facts, when fiber enters the body it combines with water and forms a "gel-like substance" in the stomach. This gel-like substance slows down and reduces insulin spikes.

By focusing on the consumption of high fiber foods, combined with the other Perfect Detox core principles, it may lead to lower a1c numbers.

9. **How will I know if the detox is working?**

    First, you could check your labs. Have they improved from your last set of blood work tests? Second, there's the weight scale. Have you seen any fluctuations in weight throughout the 10 days?

    Third, there's your measurements. Have you lost inches off your waist, arms, and/or legs since the beginning of the program?

    Lastly, and more importantly, how do you feel? More energized? Less brain fog? Better about yourself in general?

10. **What type of supplies or equipment do I need for the detox?**

    Keep in mind, that most of these items are optional. What you will need will be based on what type of foods and drinks you plan to consume.

    Next to each item, I've included some samples of what that item would be useful for during the program (and after).

1. Blender – Smoothies. Smoothie Bowls.
2. Juicer – Fresh Juices.
3. Cutting Knives – Dicing, chopping, and preparing fruits and vegetables.
4. Cutting Board – For dicing and cutting (prepping) fruits and vegetables.
5. Storage Containers – Vegetable meals, prepped fruit, herbs, and prepped vegetables.
6. Tea Strainer – To strain loose-leaf tea.
7. Juice Strainer – To strain excess foam/pulp as you juice.
8. Mason Jars – To store fresh pressed juice, smoothies, prepped fruit, and prepped vegetables.
9. Ziploc Bags – For freezing and storing bananas. Frozen bananas can be used to make nice cream (see recipe section), and creamy/cold smoothies.
    a. Great for allowing vegetables to marinate in balsamic vinegar and seasonings.
    b. Can be used to bring fruit to snack on throughout the day.
10. Food Processor – for use in making plant-based meats, desserts, dips, and chopping.

11. How do I best store fruits and vegetables so they stay fresh longer?

PRODUCE STORAGE TIPS

Refrigerator

apples, pears
beets, turnips
berries, cherrries, grapes
broccolli, cauliflower
lettuce, leafy greens
cucumber, corn, eggplant, peppers
zucchini, fresh herbs

Counter and Pantry

bananas, citrus fruits, avocado, melons,
peaches, garlic, onions
watermelon, hard Squash

12. Will I lose belly fat with this detox?

You cannot "spot reduce" or "spot specific" weight loss efforts. Typically, weight loss happens in the following order:

1st The face

2nd The chest

3rd The hips and butt

4th The abdominal area

13. **Can I consume nut and seed butter (peanut butter, almond butter, etc.)?**

    No, these kinds of butter are high in fat. They are also sometimes produced with oils. These are not ideal to consume during cleanse.

14. **Can I consume veggies that have been cooked with meat or animal broth?**

    No, animal sources of protein or liquids can be consumed.

15. **What can I do if I am experiencing low energy?**

    1. Rest
    2. Eat bananas and/or dates. They are both great for quick energy. You can consume them as is or make a smoothie and put them in it.
    3. Stay hydrated. If necessary, you can put a few sprinkles, of "no sugar added" electrolytes in your water.

16. **Can I follow The Perfect 10 Detox long-term?**

    No. This is not a sustainable way of eating long-term. You should never use a method that eliminates entire food group as a sustainable way to eat.

17. **I do intense exercise, any pre-workout recommendations that aid with workout endurance and hydration?**

    - Eat a banana or large apple 15-30 minutes before a heavier workout. Then eat a banana or large apple after your workout.

- If you are in phase 1 or 2 of the program, increase our intake of chickpeas. These are higher calorie than fruits and vegetables.
- If in phase 2, take advantage of being able to consume avocado.
- Enjoy fresh fruit juice before your workout and during. Fresh fruit juice contains natural sugars which serve as a natural energy booster.

18. **Why do some of the recipes only have ingredients listed versus the measurements for how much to add?**

   Short answer, if you do not like it, you will not enjoy it, which means you will not consume it for 10 days. Making healthy food that you enjoy is the secret to a successful cleanse.

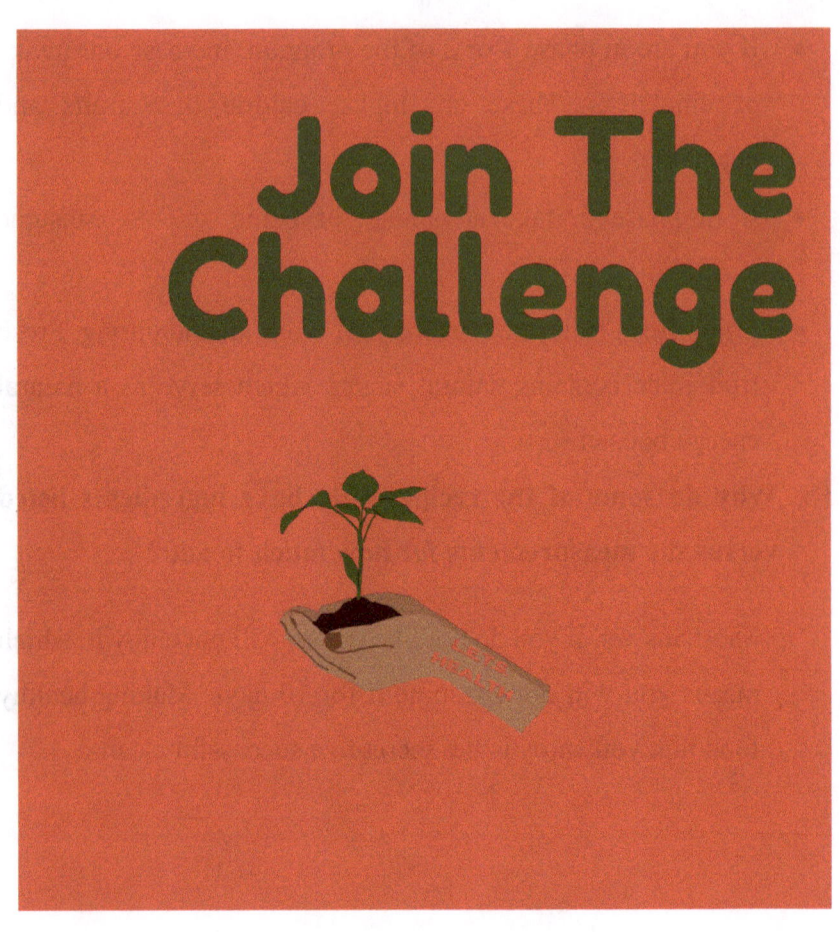

Chapter 11

Join The Challenge

Now that you know about The Perfect 10 Detox. It's time for you to join the challenge!

I host a monthly detox group on Facebook. It is a private group where only those who register via my website (letshealth.biz) can access the community and information.

Here is why you should join:

1. Joining the group offers accountability, support, and questions quickly answered throughout the challenge.
2. You get to navigate the challenges of the detox with me and "the community" by your side.

The simple truth is that most people are more likely to succeed with support and accountability. Participants have transformed their health, cognitive abilities, weight, and their mindset during the Perfect 10 Detox.

If you are still apprehensive about the need and benefits of cleansing, I don't know what to tell you. The choice is yours and results don't lie.

Many of us are a ticking time bomb for health issues. On the surface you may feel fine, feel like you are managing your symptoms, "good enough", but ultimately it all catches up to us.

Think about what happened to me in 2022. I weighed 180ish pounds, standing at only 5'7". I was fluctuating between processed junk foods, fasting, vegan eating, excessive caffeine, and processed animal-based protein consumption. You see with the plant-based/vegan diet becoming so popular and very much in demand, processed vegan options began popping up everywhere. These vegan foods, although very convenient, were not considered "whole foods". I fell into this style of eating more and more until being a junk food vegan was a more fitting category for me. That is where weight gain, high cholesterol, sluggishness, emotional eating, and just an overall unhealthy way of living blossomed.

But I was "seemingly fine".

If that was not enough, both the suppressed stress (and grief) due to losing a loved one and the daily stress I was enduring for months leading up to that day was off the charts. I was battling anxiety and didn't even realize it.

But the bottom line was my body had had enough! It had just chosen that day in April 2022 to reveal itself. But I thank God for his faithfulness, for providing fruits and vegetables (and the knowledge of how to use them), and the chance to improve my quality of life.

This DETOX is for you!

Join The Challenge!

Recipes, Food Ideas, and Tips

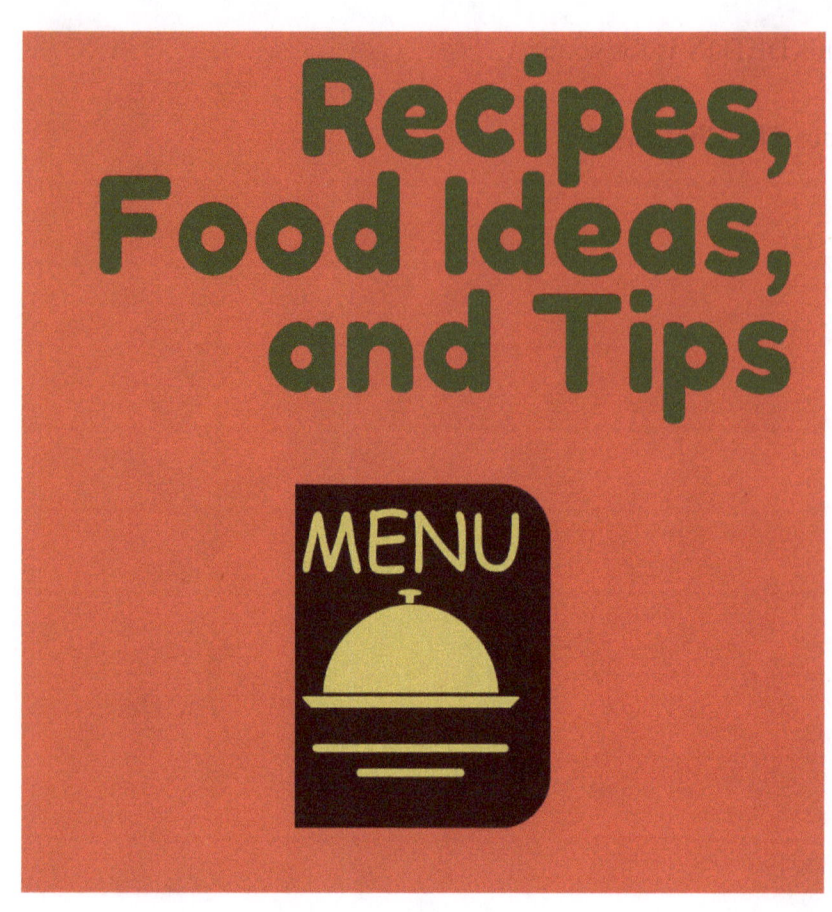

Chapter 12

Recipes, Food Ideas, and Tips

The + sign means you can consume that recipe during that particular phase of the detox.

The x sign means you cannot consume that recipe during that particular phase of the detox.

	Recipe	Phase 1	Phase 2	Phase 3
	Juices			
1	Perfect Detox Juice	+	+	+
2	Herbal Drink	+	+	+
3	Citrus Kickstarter Juice	+	+	+
4	Wonderful Watermelon Juice	+	+	+
5	Anti-Inflammatory Juice	+	+	+
6	Constipation Crusher Juice	+	+	+
	Arthritis Away Juice	+	+	+
7	Hypertension Healer Juice	+	+	+
	Allergy Avenger Juice	+	+	+
8	Awesome Arteries Juice	+	+	+
	Lung Support Juice	+	+	+
9	Heart Healthy Juice	+	+	+
	Smoothies			
10	Berry Crazy Smoothie	+	+	+
11	Let's Get Tropical Smoothie	+	+	+
12	Green Machine Smoothie	+	+	+
	Fruits			
13	Fruit Cereal	+	+	+
14	Tomato Cucumber Peppers Avocado (TCPA) Salad	no avocado	+	no avocado

15	Southern Mango Salad	+	+	+
16	Berry Fruity Nice Cream	+	+	+
17	Avocado Zucchini Noodles	X	+	X
Sauces, Dips, and Dressings				
18	L.E.T.S. Health 1-2-3 Dressing	+	+	+
19	Chickpea Hummus	+	+	X
20	Get Limey Dressing	+	+	+
21	Guacamole	X	+	X
22	Dates Sauce	X	+	+
Vegetables				
23	Phase 1 Veggie Meal Prep	+	X	X
24	Cabbage + Veggies Soup	+	X	X
25	Veggie Wraps	+	+	+

Juicing Tips

Juicing is a great way to detoxify the body through the elimination pathways. It does require some tools to get started, and a little know-how to operate and get the most high-quality juice from a juicer. Don't let any of that intimidate you away from juicing. Once you get into it, it is quite simple. When it comes to what equipment you need to start juicing with, you have the option of using a juicer or a combination of a nut bag and a blender.

There are 2 main types of juicers:

1. Cold Press Juicer
2. Masticating Juicers

Cold press juicers are going to yield a higher quality of juice. It is a slower juicer so it "squeezes" out more juice from the produce. Cold press juicers tend to be more expensive than most juicers.

Masticating juicers juice faster than cold press juicers. They tend to be less expensive than cold press juicers. Most masticating juicers will not "squeeze" every drip out of your produce, results in more money being spent on fruits and vegetables to produce more juice.

Other helpful juicing equipment will include:

1. Juice strainer – a juice strainer is used to remove foam and pulp from your juice.
2. Glass jars – glass jars are used with tops to store your juice.
3. Knives/cutting boards- knives and cutting boards are used to prep your fruits and vegetables for juicing and/or blending.
4. Nut bag- a nut bag is used to strain juice pulp if you are using a blender.

Directions to use blender for juice:

1. Clean and prep your fruits and/or your vegetables.
2. If not organic, peel off the skin.
3. If skin is very tough, peel off the skin.
    a. For example, watermelons, cantaloupes, and pineapples.
4. Put fruit and vegetables in blender. If they are not juicy fruits or if they are leafy greens, add some water to the blender before blending.

5. Blend until well blended, then strain into a container with a nut bag or juice strainer.

Ultimately, buy what your budget can afford, even if it's a masticating juicer, you will still get great results.

These are some of my favorite juices for healing. I did not list quantities of each ingredient for every recipe because I am a firm believer in how you must adapt your juice to your taste buds. If it's disgusting or you don't like it, you are less likely to be consistent with consumption.

Juices

1

The Perfect Detox Juice

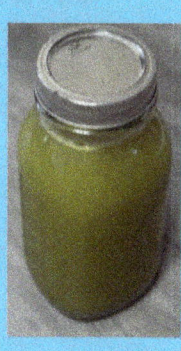
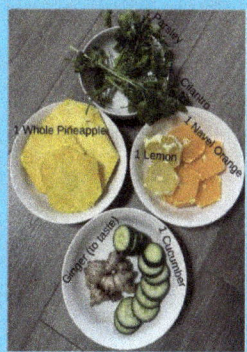

- **Cilantro** – helps remove metals such as mercury, lead, and aluminum from the body.
- **Parsley** – stimulates the release of bile, which helps the liver detox.
- **Ginger** – fights germs, illness, and inflammation. Stimulates digestion, sweating, and circulation which aids in elimination.
- **Pineapple** – may reduce the risk of high cholesterol (LDL).
- **Orange** – the high water content helps flush toxins from the body through urine. Also a great source of Vitamin C.
- **Lemon** – helps support the liver in production of bile to move food smoothly through the intestinal tract. It is also great for the skin.
- **Cucumbers** – good for healthy skin, bone health, muscle function, great source of antioxidants and may help with cancer prevention.

2

Herbal Green Drink

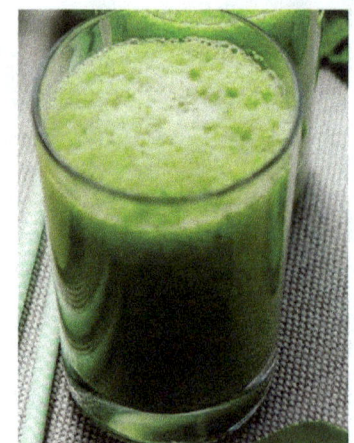

Ingredients (to taste)
- Cilantro
- Parsley
- Ginger
- Lemon or Lime or Both

Directions
- Blend it or Juice it
- Serve chilled

3

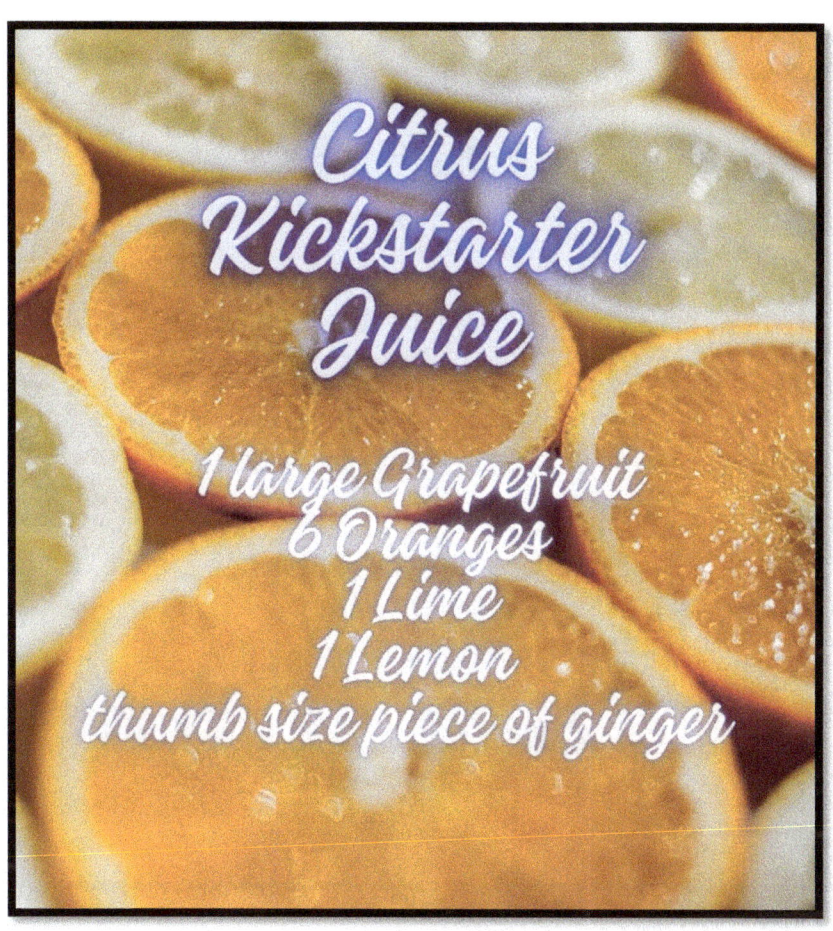

Citrus Kickstarter Juice

1 large Grapefruit
6 Oranges
1 Lime
1 Lemon
thumb size piece of ginger

4

Wonderful Watermelon

WATERMELON
LIMES
CILANTRO
PARSLEY
GINGER

(TO TASTE)

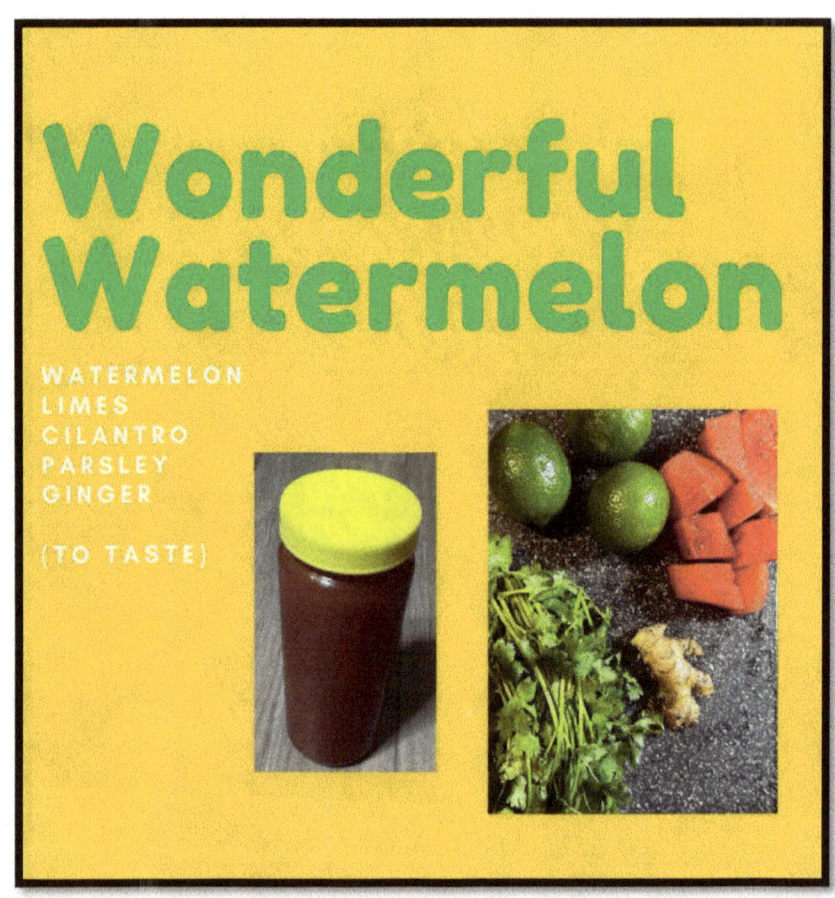

5

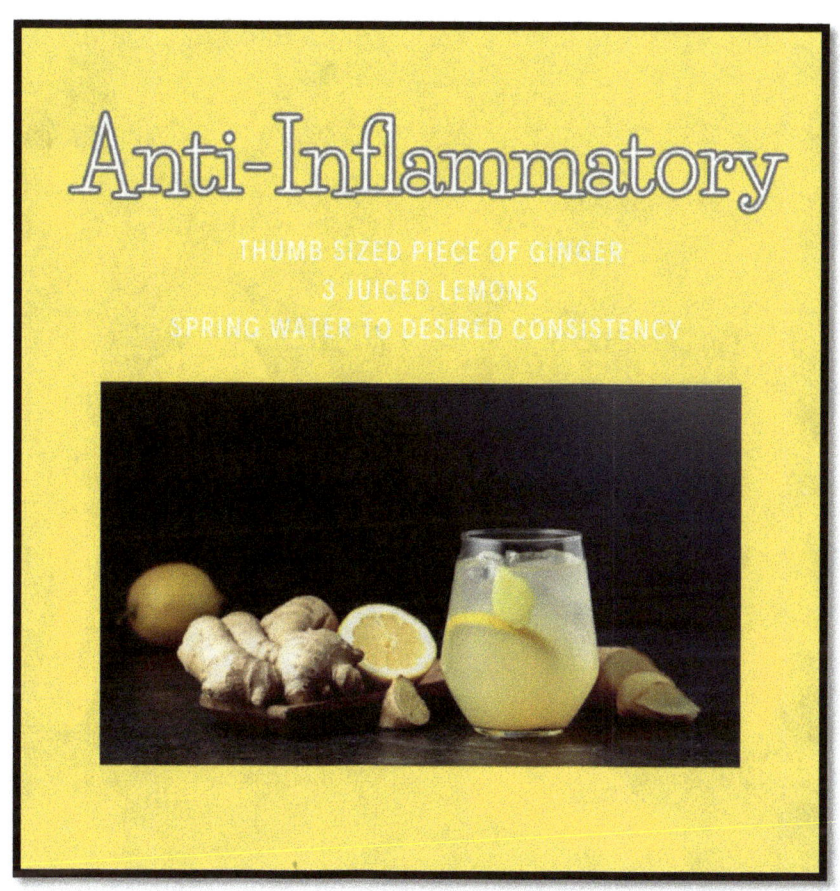

Anti-Inflammatory

THUMB SIZED PIECE OF GINGER
3 JUICED LEMONS
SPRING WATER TO DESIRED CONSISTENCY

6

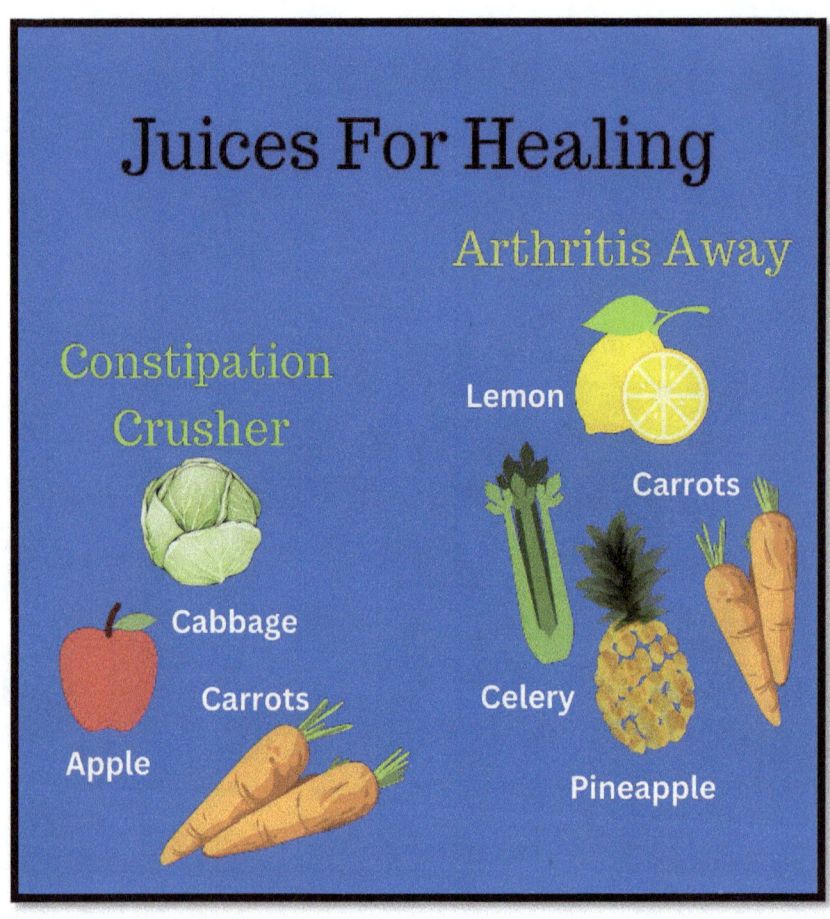

7

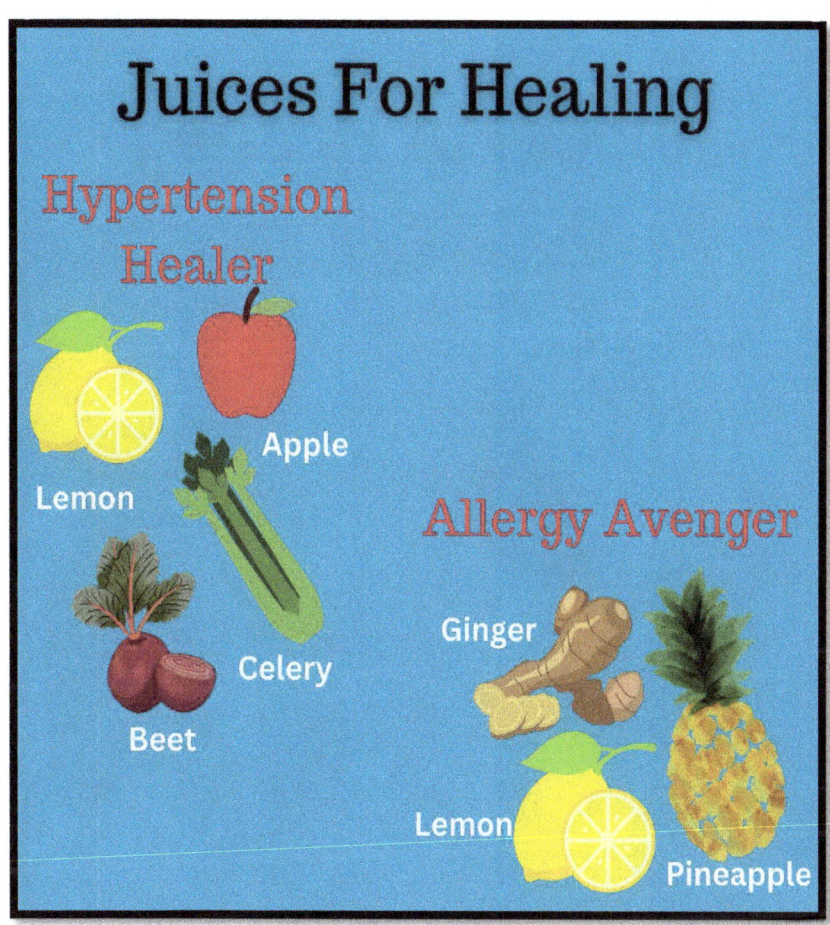

8

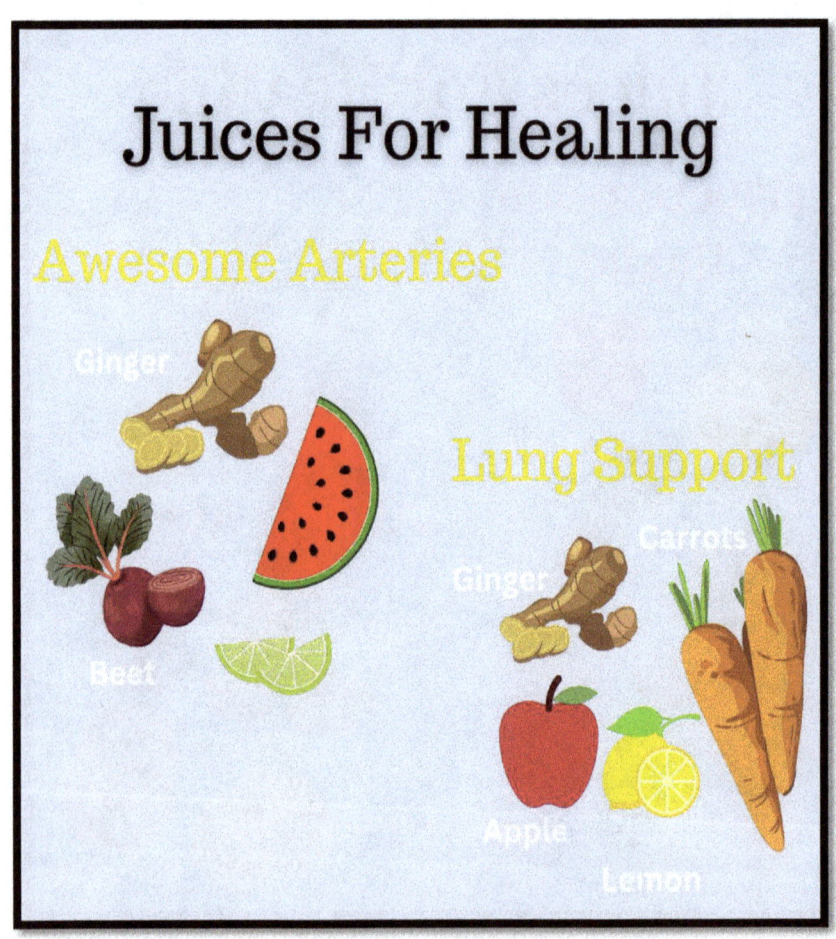

9

Heart Healthy

Apples
Beets
Ginger
Lemon

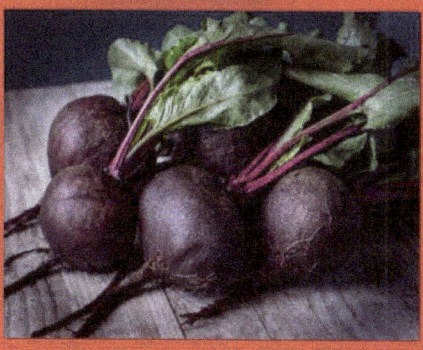

The quantity of each ingredient should fit your taste buds

Smoothie Tips

1. Smoothies are a great way to consume your fruits and vegetables while still benefiting from their fiber. Smoothies also are a great option for those who may not like the taste of vegetables. By combining them with your favorite fruits, you can consume way more nutrients in a portable way.

2. Use both frozen fruit and fresh fruit when possible. That way, you do not have to add ice to make it cold. Plus, frozen fruits last longer than fresh (from spoiling).

3. Use fruits and vegetables that you enjoy. Stick to the "80/20" rule (80% fruits and 20% vegetables) until you develop a taste for more vegetable/greens-based smoothies.

4. For the purposes of this detox program, do not add any fats to your smoothies.

Smoothies

10

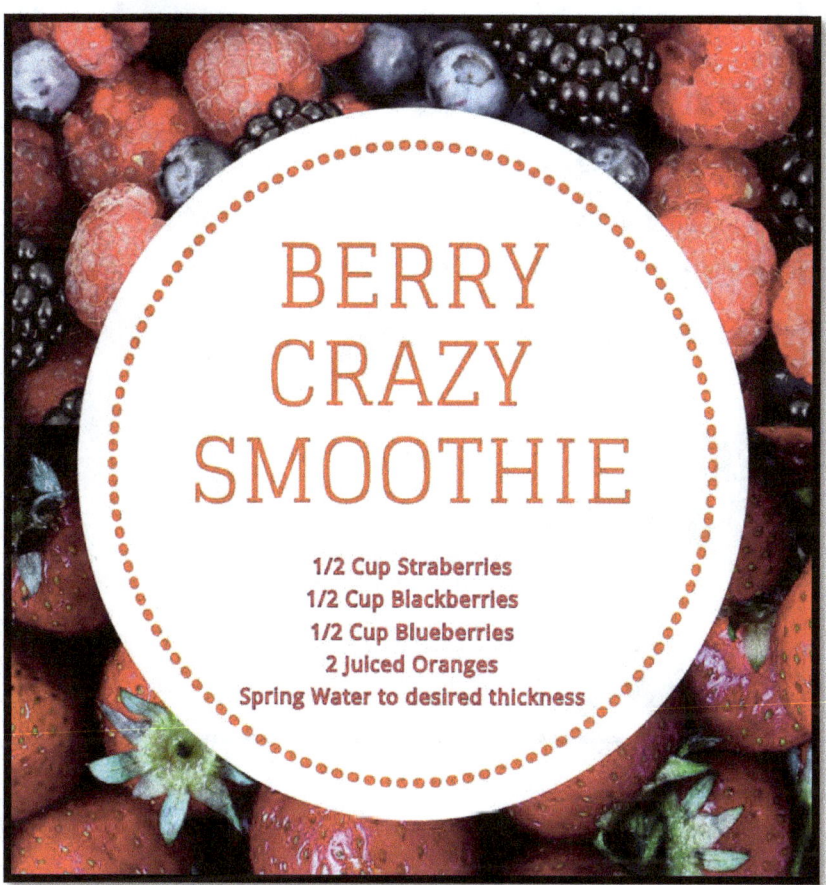

BERRY CRAZY SMOOTHIE

1/2 Cup Straberries
1/2 Cup Blackberries
1/2 Cup Blueberries
2 Juiced Oranges
Spring Water to desired thickness

11

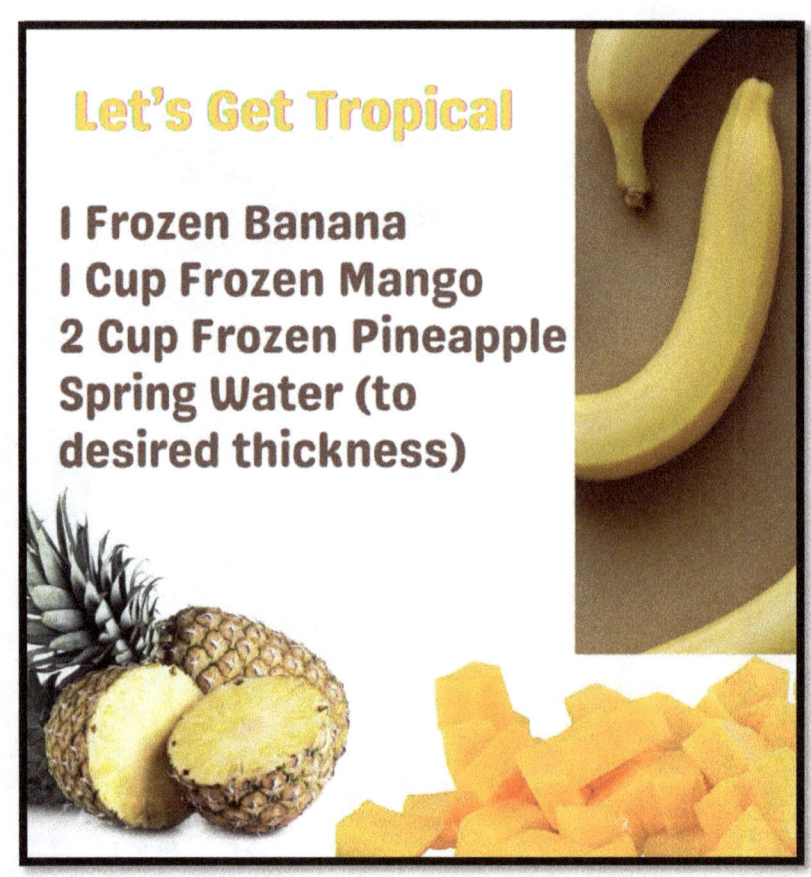

Let's Get Tropical

1 Frozen Banana
1 Cup Frozen Mango
2 Cup Frozen Pineapple
Spring Water (to desired thickness)

Green Machine Smoothie

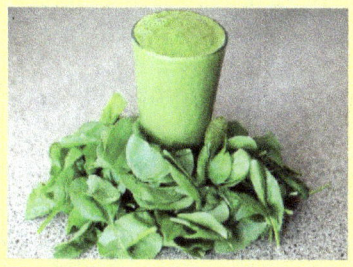 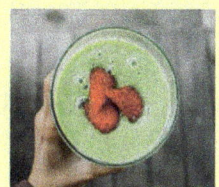

Ingredients:
- 1 Frozen Banana
- 1 Cup Strawberry
- 2-3 Handfuls of Baby Spinach
- ½ Tablespoon Cinnamon
- Unsweetened Plant Milk (almond milk, cashew milk) - to your desired thickness (start with 1 cup and then add more to your desired thickness)

Directions:
- Combine all ingredients in blender.
- Add in additional plant milk (to desired consistency)

Fruit and Vegetable Snacking Tips

1. Prepare your fruit in advance. Have it already cleaned, peeled, and put into containers or baggies. That way, when you are ready to snack, your fruit is ready too.

2. When you are travelling or hanging out, bring fruit with protective layers such as bananas, oranges, apples, or pears. This way you do not need containers or need access to water to clean the fruit.

3. Always overpack. Until you have determined how much fruit and vegetables you will need or consume on a given day, it is better to bring more than enough.

4. To ensure that you do not waste money on produce that goes bad before you have the time to eat it, do not buy too much at any one time. Plan to visit the grocery store or local market every 2-3 days.

5. Apples or bananas are a great pre- and post-workout snack. If you're into fitness activities, keep one with you.

Fruits

13

Fruit Cereal

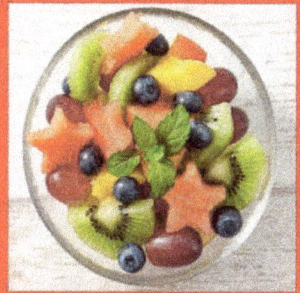 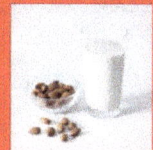

Ingredients:
- Any fruit that you like
- Unsweetened almond milk or other unsweetened nut milk

Directions:
- Wash and prepare your fruit
- Once you've prepared all your fruit, place the fruit into a bowl
- Pour some chilled, non-dairy milk overtop and enjoy!

14

Tomato Cucumber Peppers Avocado salad (TCPA)

Dice and combine with
Balsamic Vinegar and No salt Seasonings or 1-2-3 dressing
Date Syrup or Maple Syrup (optional)

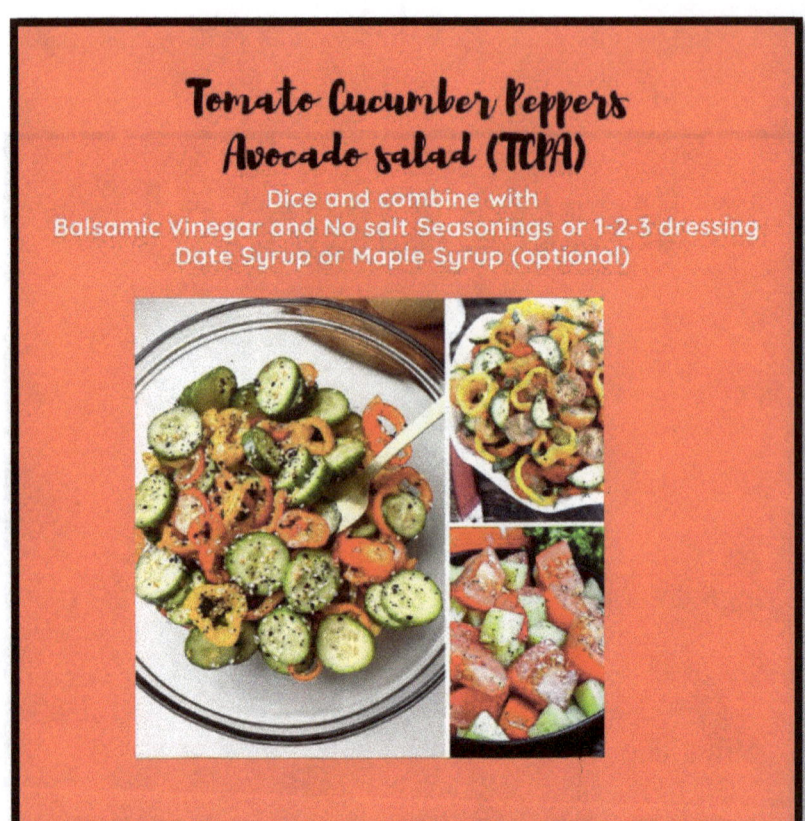

15

Southern Mango Salad

Ingredients
- Diced Mangos
- Diced Red bell pepper
- Sliced or diced Cucumber
- sliced or diced Red onion
- Fresh mint
- Fresh cilantro

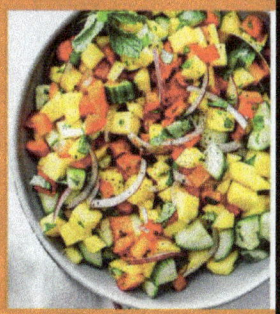

Dressing
- Lime juice - 2 limes juiced
- Maple or Dates syrup - 1 tablespoon
- Salt free seasoning - (optional)

16

Berry Fruity Smoothie Bowl

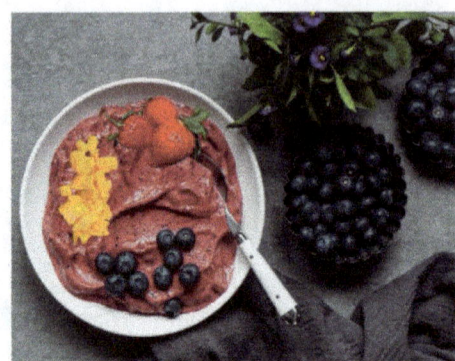

Ingredients:
- Frozen Banana(s)
- Berries
- Cinnamon
- Unsweetened plant milk (almond milk, cashew milk) -add in last to your desired thickness

Directions:
- Combine all ingredients in blender or processor
- slowly add in plant milk to desired consistency
- Top with any fruit of choice

Avocado Zucchini Noodles

Ingredients

- 2-3 zucchini
- 1 avocado
- 1/4 cup fresh lime juice (about 2 limes)
- 3/4 cup water or vegetable broth
- 1 teaspoon sea salt (optional)
- 1 teaspoon black pepper
- 1 teaspoon garlic powder (optional)

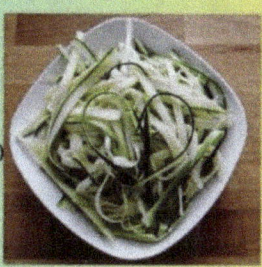

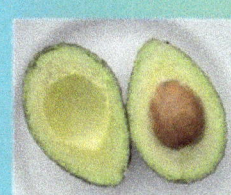

Directions

- Place all ingredients, except the zuchinni, in a blender and blend until smooth.
- Use a spiralizer to turn your zuchinni into noodles.
- Place your noodles on a plate or in large bowl. Pour the avocado mixture ontop the noodles.
- Top with diced tomato, mushrooms, or any other non-starchy vegetables that you enjoy.

Sauces, Dips, and Dressings

18

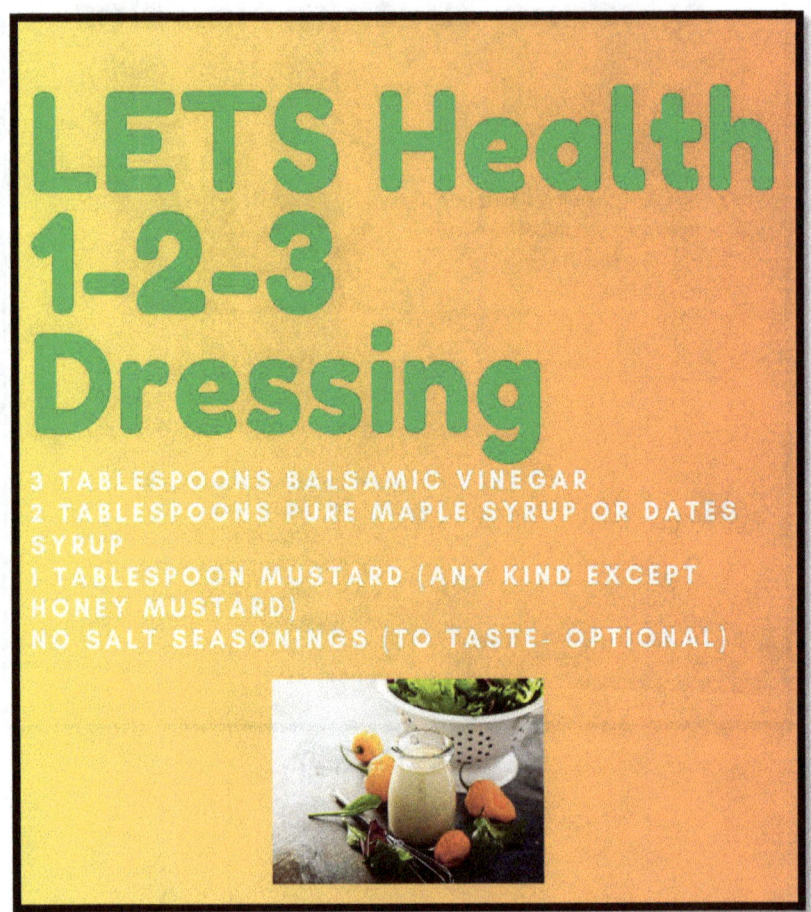

LETS Health 1-2-3 Dressing

3 TABLESPOONS BALSAMIC VINEGAR
2 TABLESPOONS PURE MAPLE SYRUP OR DATES SYRUP
1 TABLESPOON MUSTARD (ANY KIND EXCEPT HONEY MUSTARD)
NO SALT SEASONINGS (TO TASTE- OPTIONAL)

19

Chickpea Hummus

Ingredients
- 1 - 15 oz can of chickpeas (or 2 cups of cooked chickpeas)
- 4 cloves of garlic or garlic powder to taste
- 1 squeezed lemon or 1/4 cup lemon juice
- 1/4 to 1/2 cup balsamic vinegar and chickpea liquid from can (to desired consistency)

Optional
- crushed red pepers
- onions
- salt free seasonings

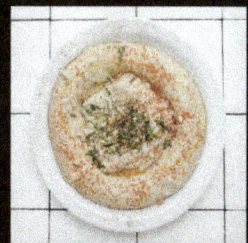

Directions
- combine all ingredients into a blender or food processor
- blend till desired consistency
- store in a airtight container.

Get Limey Dressing

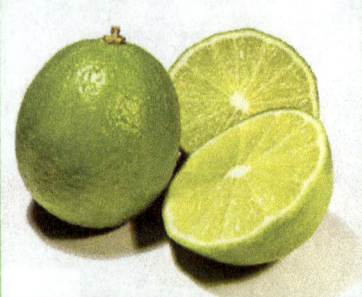

Ingredients:
- 1/2 cup aquafaba (liquid from a can of no-salt-added chickpeas)
- 1/4 cup fresh lime juice (use fresh for best flavor, but bottled can be used)
- 1-2 pitted Medjool dates (for sweetness, adjust to taste)
- 1 tablespoon balsamic vinegar
- 1/2 teaspoon minced garlic or 1 teaspoon garlic powder
- 1/8 teaspoon fresh cracked black pepper
- 1/2 teaspoon cilantro
- ¼ avocado (only during phase 2)

Directions:
Place wet ingredients in blender or food processor, combine.
Then add in dry ingriedients and combine fully.

Guacamole

Ingredients

- 1 Medium Ripe Avocados
- 1/2 Cup Green Peas
- 1 teaspoon garlic powder
- 1 teaspoon onion powder
- ½ teaspoon freshly ground black pepper
- 1-2 Tablespoons lime juice
- 2 Tablespoons chopped fresh cilantro
- 1 small tomatoes diced
- ½ teaspoon cayenne pepper, or jalapeno pepper diced (optional)

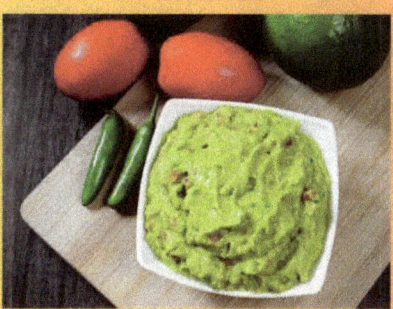

Directions

- Add all ingredients accept the avocado to a food processor blender.
- Process the vegetables and seasonings
- Add avocado to bowl and mash well.
- Add in the mixture from the food processor or blender.

22

Dates Sauce

Ingredients:
- 2 cup medjool dates
- Water

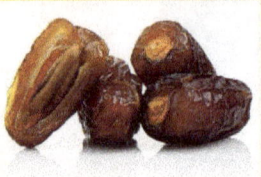

Directions:
1. Cover the pitted dates with water and leave it soaking for 2-4 hours in a bowl.
2. Place the pitted dates and the soaking water in a blender. Blend until a smooth paste is formed (time will vary depending on what dates you're using and blender wattage)
3. Keep in on the fridge and use it instead of sweetners.

Vegetables Tips

- Until you have determined how much vegetables you will need or consume on a given day, it is better to have more than enough.

- To ensure that you do not waste money on produce that goes bad before you have time to eat it, do not buy too much at any one time. Plan to visit the grocery store or market every 2-3 days.

<u>Vegetables</u>

23

PHASE I VEGGIE MEAL PREP TIP

STEP 1 BUY A BIG BAG OF FROZEN VEGGIES
STEP 2 PORTION THE BAG INTO GLASS OR PLASTIC CONTAINERS

WHEN YOU YOU ARE READY TO EAT

STEP 3 SAUTEE FRESH DICED ONIONS, MUSHROOMS, AND PEPPERS WITH NO SALT SEASONINGS

STEP 4 WARM THE FROZEN VEGGIES UP IN MICRO AND DRAIN ANY EXCESS WATER.

STEP 5 ADD IN SAUTEED VEGGIES

STEP 6 AT MORE NO SALT SEASONINGS OR CONDIMENTS TO TASTE

STEP 7 ENJOY!

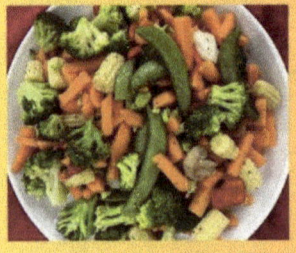 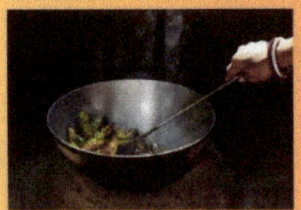

24

Cabbage + Veggies Soup

- **Mushrooms - Any Kind**
- **Low Sodium Vegetable Broth**
- **Diced Bell Peppers (red, yellow, green)**
- **Onions - Any Kind**
- **Carrots**
- **Okra**
- **Cabbage**
- **Cauliflower Rice**

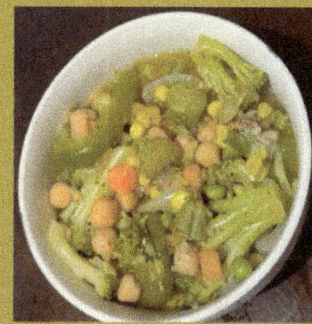

The non starchy vegetables of your choice- can be fresh or frozen)

25

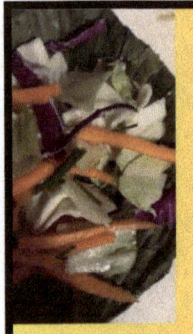

Veggie Wraps

Wrap Ideas:
- Collard Greens
- Romaine Lettuce
- Dehydrated Wraps

Fill It With:
- onions
- peppers
- mushrooms
- tomato
- cucumber
- any non-starchy vegetables

Sauces: balsamic vinegar, maple syrup, mustard, fat free italian, 1-2-3 Dressing, go limey dressing, oil free hummus

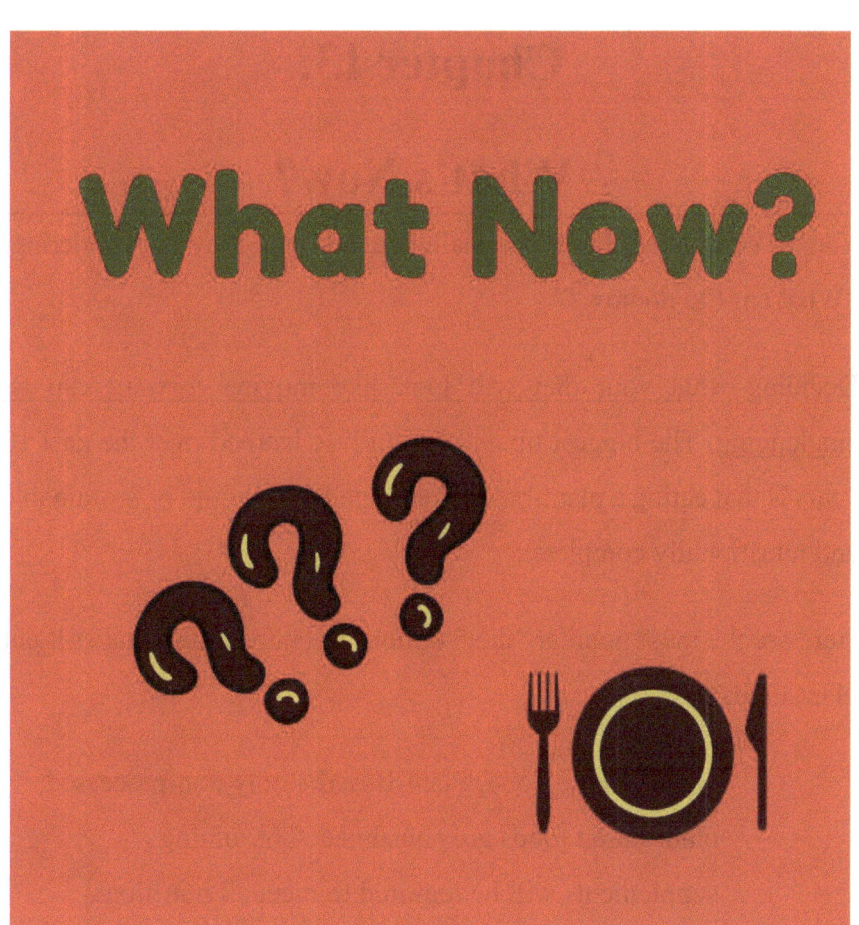

Chapter 13:

What's Now?

You've completed the detox challenge, and you may be wondering, "What am I to do now?"

Deciding <u>what your diet will look like moving forward can be challenging</u>. The biggest tip and lesson I've learned over the past 10 years is that eating a plant-based dominated diet should be sustainable and nutritionally complete.

Here are the most popular "diet" options to choose from that still put plant foods first:

1. 100% Whole Food, Plant-Based – only non-processed, plant-based foods are consumed. Consuming supplements will be required to meet all nutritional needs.
2. Mostly Whole Food, Plant-Based – majority of diet is focused on whole plant foods, with the consumption of some unprocessed animal sources of protein (less than 15 percent of diet).
3. Vegetarian – a diet consisting of plant-based foods, as well as dairy, eggs, and honey. This diet does not include fish, seafood, red meat, or poultry.

4. Pescatarian – a diet consisting of the same food options as a vegetarian diet but also allows fish and seafood. This diet does not include eating red meat or poultry.
5. Polo-Pescatarian – this diet follows all the same guidelines as a pescatarian diet and adds poultry consumption to the diet.

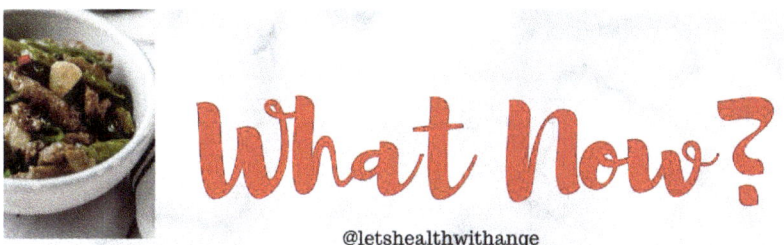

@letshealthwithange

Reintroducing foods after your Cleanse

- Leafy Green Vegetables
- Non-Starchy Vegetables
- Beans and Chickpeas
- Sweet Potatoes, Quinoa, Brown Rice
- Lean Protein (if you plan to consume meat) - cod fish, flounder, haddock, shrimp, tuna, egg whites (air fry, bake, broil, no breading or coating, do not fry)
- Tofu and Tempeh
- Continue eating fruit (2-4 servings per day)
- Maintain a low fat diet consisting of whole non-processed foods
- Avoid Oils
- Limit Salt Intake
- Limit Added Sugars

@LETSHealthWithAnge

150

Transitioning back to "other foods" after the detox:

1. Keep your consumption of whole, plant foods going. Continue eating the foods you enjoyed during phases 1, 2, and 3 of the program.
2. Depending on what style of eating you plan to eat going forward, these are some samples of transition foods to integrate into your daily diet over the next 3-5 days.

Sweet Potato	Lean Sources of Protein (with 1 meal per day)	Quinoa
Brown Rice	Whole Oats	Beans – any kind

After 3-5 days, you can start integrating more lean sources of protein with more meals per day. Listen to your body. If it causes digestive issues or discomfort, don't eat it.

Examples of 100% plant-based friendly foods you can consume after the detox as you transition back to other foods.

- Oatmeal with cinnamon, banana, and apples
- Cooked veggies with chickpeas
- Whole grain or sprouted bread with chickpea humus, lettuce tomato, and mushrooms
- Baked sweet potato fries

- Quinoa topped with seasoned black beans and salsa

Examples of Vegetarian/pescatarian-friendly foods for after the detox as you transition back to other foods

- Egg whites with spinach and veggies scrambled
- Cooked cabbage soup with baked cod
- Protein shake with fruit
- Greek yogurt bowl with fruit and topped with grape nuts

Next Month (The month after your detox)

If your goals have not been met, complete The Perfect 10 Detox program again. You can choose to start back over with Phase 1 and then progress to phase 3, or begin at any phase you feel comfortable with. At this point, it's up to you and your needs.

If your goals were met, CONGRATS! You now have all the tools to do this program any time you need to.

When deciding what type of diet is sustainable and fulfilling for you moving forward, do some research and learning on your own. The best way to dive into all the benefits and studies is to read books and watch relevant documentaries.

Here is a list of some of my favorite books:

- Dr. Neal Barnard's Program for Reversing Diabetes: The Scientifically Proven System for Reversing Diabetes by Dr. Neal D. Barnard, M.D.

- How To Eat Plant-based Like a Boss by Angela Bentley-Henry, M.Ed.

- Got Sea Moss? The Beginner's Guide to the Ultimate Supplement by Angela Bentley-Henry, M.Ed.

- I Love to Jump Rope: A Jump Roping Handbook for Better Fitness and Health by Angela Bentley-Henry, M.Ed.

- The Engine 2 Seven-Day Rescue Diet: Eat Plants, Lose Weight, Save Your Health by Rip Esselstyn

- Mucusless Diet Healing System by Arnold Ehret

Not much of a reader? Or simply like to supplement your reading with documentaries? Here are some great informative documentaries:

- Forks Over Knives

- Feel Rich
- What The Health?
- Fat, Sick, and Nearly Dead
- Game Changers

These resources will help you map out your diet going forward.

Good luck! You got this! Your journey to ideal health is already in motion.

Please keep in touch, I'd love to hear about your successes along the way.

About The Author

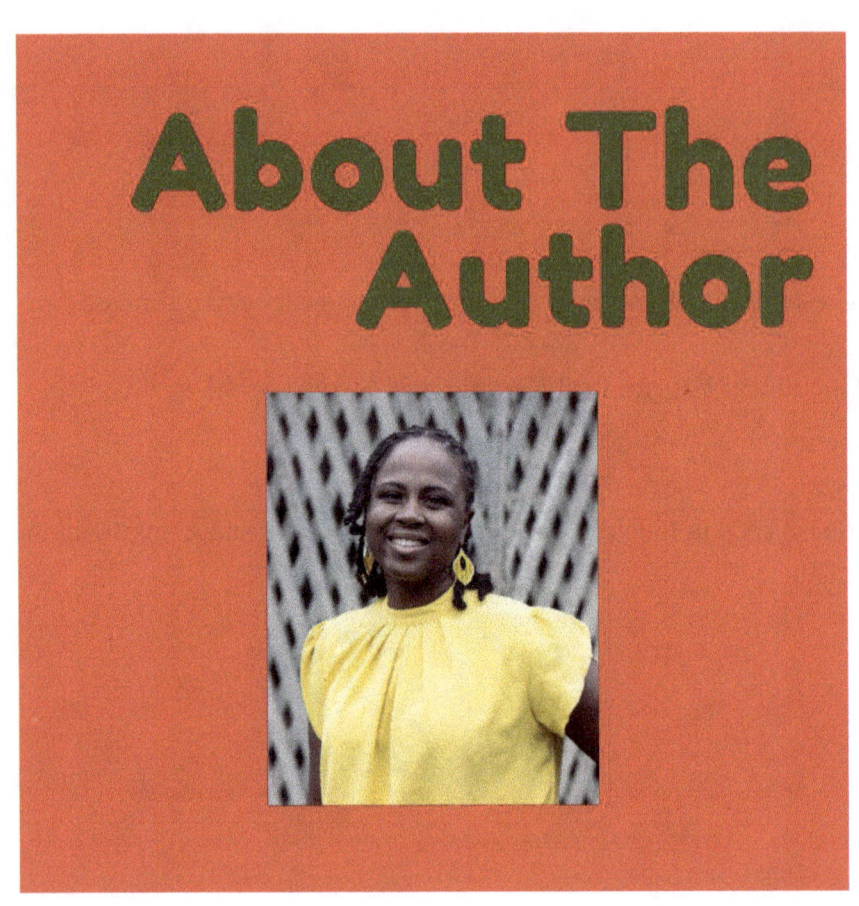

About The Author

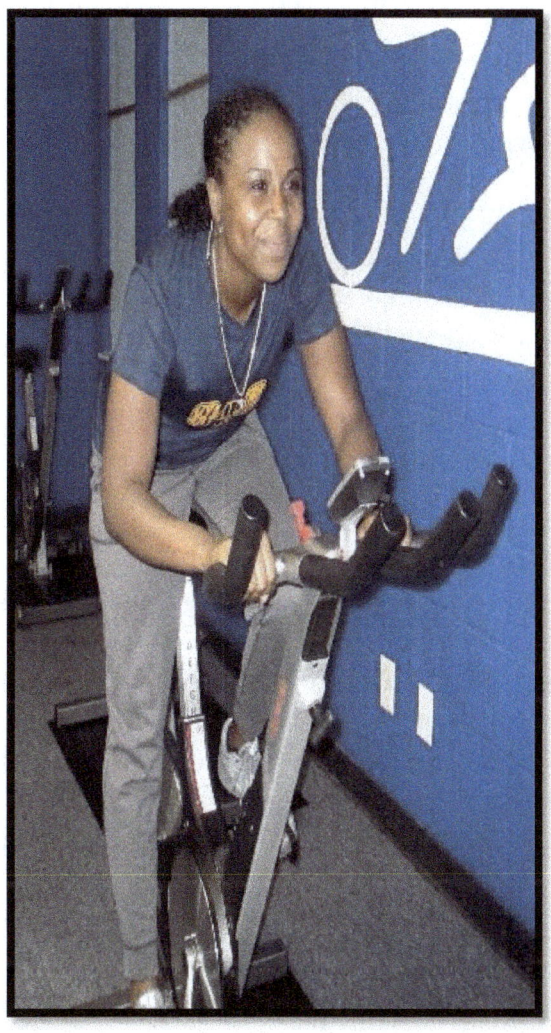

Educating and inspiring others to eat plant-based and live healthy and fit lifestyles is truly Angela's passion. Seeing others benefit from plant-based eating combined with physical activity is a personal mission that she has taken on since the death of her grandmother. Angela watched her grandmother fight a 20-year battle with diabetes (which led to strokes, feeding tubes, being wheelchair-bound, and needing a pacemaker). Before her grandmother's death, Angela did not know that there was a way to battle diabetes, hypertension, and other lifestyle diseases. In 2022, when an abnormal EKG led to her having to see a cardiologist. She now believes in the power of plants. Her life has been the proof.

Angela grew up in a small town where healthy options weren't always available. She was very active throughout her childhood and teenage years. Angela played sports in school and was a standout basketball player. After college, she even had the opportunity to play semi-professional basketball. Because of her active lifestyle, Angela appeared to be very healthy. She did not have any bodyweight issues and, thus, saw no reason to change the way she ate (which wasn't very plant-based). However, over time, those unhealthy eating habits caught up with her. In 2015 (the same year her grandmother passed away), Angela was diagnosed with pre-diabetes and was severely overweight.

She truly understands the desire a person has to live healthily while enjoying the foods they are eating. Loving the food she is eating, and recreating those foods in delicious and creative ways, has always been fun and important to her. Throughout her childhood and teenage years, Angela spent most weeknights and weekends experimenting with recipes in the kitchen with her mom and watching the Food Network. This same pleasure of cooking continues throughout her plant-based journey. Sharing delicious recipes with others brings her joy.

Plant-based eating is the reason why Angela has lost over 50 pounds and reversed her pre-diabetes. It is also how she is living a healthier, higher-quality life. By sharing the benefits of plant-based eating with others, as well as providing tips and suggestions for navigating the day-to-day experiences of eating plant-based, she wishes to improve the quality of life for many.

Angela truly believes that plants provide her with the fuel she needs to engage in activities she loves, like playing basketball, staying busy with her daughters, jumping rope, and working out. Angela hopes to inspire others to fuel their lives with plants as well.

Degrees:

- Master of Science in Education – Nova Southeastern University
- Graduate Certificate Nutrition (In Progress) -- Liberty University
- Bachelor of Science – University of Central Florida
- Associates Degree – University of South Florida

Certifications:

- Plant-based Cooking – Rouxbe, Forks Over Knives
- Health Education – Florida Department of Education
- Physical Education – Florida Department of Education
- Weight Management Specialist – The National Council for Certified Personal Trainers
- Punk Rope Jump Rope Instructor – Punk Rope, Inc.

Professional:

- Physical Education and Health Teacher
- Track and Field Coach
- Other Sports Coached: Soccer and Basketball
- Brevard Public School, Healthy Liaison (School Based)
- Supplements Provider (Sea Moss, Bladderwrack, Shilajit, Herbal Tea)
- Life Insurance and Annuity Agent (Florida certified)

Publications and Resources:

- Author, "How to Eat Plant-based Like A Boss"

- Author, "Got Sea Moss? The Beginner's Guide to The Ultimate Supplement"

- I Love to Jump Rope: A Jump Roping Handbook for Better Fitness and Health by Angela Bentley-Henry, M.Ed.

- Author, "Level Up Your Habits: Fitness, Nutrition, and Weight Tracker: Planner, Log, and Calendar"

- Author, "Level Up Your Workouts: Fitness Journal"

- Author, "Level Up your Nutrition: Food Log"

- Supplements: Sea Moss and Bladderwrack Liquid Drops (Strawberry flavored)

All these resources and supplements can be found at https://letshealth.biz/

Citations

Watson NF, Badr MS, Belenky G, Bliwise DL, Buxton OM, Buysse D, et al. Recommended amount of sleep for a healthy adult: a joint consensus statement of the American Academy of Sleep Medicine and Sleep Research Society. *Sleep* 2015;38(6):843–844.

https://aasm.org/resources/pdf/pressroom/adult-sleep-duration-consensus.pdf [PDF – 250KB]

(https://www.cdc.gov/nchs/fastats/leading-causes-of-death.htm)

www.ingramcontent.com/pod-product-compliance
Lightning Source LLC
Chambersburg PA
CBHW060948050426
42337CB00052B/1733